MW00613791

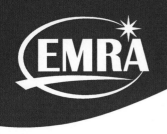

EMRA
Antibiotic Guide

20th Edition

Editor-in-Chief
Brian J. Levine, MD, FACEP
Designated Institutional Official
Associate Chief Academic Officer
Institute for Learning, Leadership & Development (iLEAD)
Department of Emergency Medicine, ChristianaCare Health System
Clinical Associate Professor of Emergency Medicine
Sidney Kimmel Medical College | Thomas Jefferson University

Associate Editors
Nicole S. Harrington, PharmD, BCPS AQ-ID
Bryan D. Hayes, PharmD, DABAT, FAACT, FASHP
Jamie M. Rosini, PharmD, MS, BCCCP, BCPS, DABAT

Senior Editors
J. Daniel Hess, MD
Jennifer Kelly, PharmD
Ramara E. Walker, PharmD, BCIDP

Assistant Editors
Jessica Beadle, MD
Elizabeth Shanahan, MD

Disclaimer

This handbook is intended as a general guide to therapy only. While the editors have taken reasonable measures to ensure the accuracy of drug and dosing information presented herein, the user should consult other resources when necessary to confirm appropriate therapy, side effects, interactions, and contraindications. The publisher, authors, editors, and sponsoring organizations specifically disclaim any liability for omissions or errors found in this handbook, for appropriate use, or treatment errors. Further, although the publisher, authors, editors, and sponsoring organizations have endeavored to make this handbook comprehensive, the vast differences in emergency practice settings may necessitate treatment approaches other than those presented here.

Copyright 2022 Emergency Medicine Residents' Association
ISBN 978-1-929854-70-7
4950 W. Royal Lane, Irving, TX 75063
972.550.0920 | **emra.org**

In Memory of Sherrill Mullenix

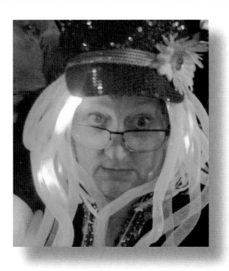

Everyone at ChristianaCare and all who knew Sherrill Mullenix were deeply saddened by the sudden loss of one of our own in January 2022.

Anyone who utilizes this book owes a debt of gratitude to Sherrill. Since the day the project was awarded to ChristianaCare, more than 10 years ago, she offered unwavering dedication and support. She was instrumental in getting the production off the ground, and she helped build this publication into the best guide in the country for emergency medicine infectious diseases. Her organization, coordination, design ideas, and determination are reflected on every page. She probably knew more about antibiotics than many of the doctors (I take that back, she definitely did)!

She displayed tenacity, spirit, and love for life. We can't thank you enough Sherrill; you made us all better for knowing you, and you are sorely missed.

- Brian Levine, MD

FOREWORD

It is a pleasure to provide you with the 2022 EMRA Antibiotic Guide. Extensive reader feedback continues to inform the format and content of the book in order to maximize its utility in the fast-paced ED environment.

The EMRA Antibiotic Guide is designed to be a quick reference, not a text on the diagnosis or comprehensive treatment of disease. The contents are organized alphabetically by organ system, followed by sections on "Special Topics" to make referencing quick and easy for a particular disease process. Abbreviations have been eliminated where possible (eg, "two times daily" as opposed to BID), and medication amounts are listed per dose, not per day. We have also attempted to simplify pediatric dosing; you will see the individual dosing for each medication that has a pediatric indication, denoted by our pediatric symbol: Ⓟ. Of special note, trimethoprim (found in TMP/SMX) dosing is based on the TMP composition. Weight-based dosing should be calculated on actual body weight — see our body weight chart.

A color-coded antibiogram lists all antibiotics from the book and the susceptibility of common organisms to each. With increasing antibiotic resistance, this section will help users to better tailor drug choices to target organisms. However, we caution to always consult local resistance data — this guide is not a substitute for such.

The medications listed are highly dependent on the editors' choices and may differ based on practice location. There may be other medications possible for individual indications that have been omitted. Pay special attention to the wording of each recommendation; unless you see "AND" or "PLUS," assume the list is a set of options from which to choose. In cases with multiple antibiotic choices, we have chosen those with the most data on efficacy or were least expensive. If the antibiotic choices were all considered equivalent, they were simply alphabetized. We have made every attempt to use specialty guidelines and peer-reviewed publications for each indication. Patient condition should be considered with each antimicrobial prescribed. In addition, consider recent (< 6 months) culture data to guide antibiotic choice. Alterations in dosing may be required for patients with renal or hepatic dysfunction.

We are deeply grateful to all those who contributed to this guide, from the faculty, residents, pharmacists, and PAs who developed the content to the experts who reviewed it. Special thanks to our pharmacy and ID gurus, **Jamie Rosini, Nicole Harrington, Ramara Walker, Jennifer Kelly**, and **Bryan Hayes** (who joined us every week from several hundred miles away). They have once again raised the bar for this edition and given countless hours to ensure its excellence, doing what they do so well: saving all of us on shift.

We hope you find this guide helpful in the care of your patients during your daily practice. We hope you continue to wonder, *"How did I survive a shift without this reference?"*

Brian J. Levine, MD, FACEP

CONTRIBUTORS

All contributors are affiliated with ChristianaCare.

Authors

BONE & JOINT
Discitis/Vertebral Osteomyelitis
Allyssa Abel, MD, MPH
Paul C. Anderson, MD
Infectious Tenosynovitis
Ryan Lee, MD
Salman Aziz, MD
Open Fracture
Douglas Ader, DO
Jeremy G. Berberian, MD
Osteomyelitis
Eric Lieu, MD
Christopher Biedrzycki, MD
Septic Arthritis
Rawaa Al Rifaie, MD
Leo Burns, MD
Septic Bursitis
Travis Kaiser Jones, DO
Leo Burns, MD

CARDIOVASCULAR
Endocarditis
Katharine Lowrey, PharmD
Michael N. Perza, PharmD

CNS
Bell's Palsy
Thomas Marconi Jr., MD
James Carroll, MD
Encephalitis
Jessica Beadle, MD
Morganne Castiglione, MD
Meningitis
Frank Mayer, DO, MBA
Valerie Cohen, DO
Spinal or Intracranial Epidural Abscess
Isaac J. Bennett, DO
Diana Cer, DO

EAR/NOSE/THROAT
ANUG
Sanjay Nadesan, MD
Lauren Cooksey, MD
Dental Abscess
Jonathan Bodner, MD
Christopher Giaquinto, PA-C
Epiglottitis
Alex Oei, DO
Julie Cooper, MD
Ludwig's Angina
Amber Higgins, MD
Dana Matelyan, PA-C
Mastoiditis
Hamna Atif, MD
Christopher Cox, MD

Otitis Externa
Brittney Bunkis, MD
Vincent Russell, PA-C
Otitis Media
Niketu Patel, MD, MPH
Vincent Russell, PA-C
Parapharyngeal Abscess
Young Daniel Cho, DO
Shivdeep Deo, MD, MS
Parotitis/Sialadenitis
Tulsi D. Patel, MD
Shivdeep Deo, MD, MS
Pertussis
Sergiu Costinas, MD
Justin Eisenman, DO, MS, FACEP, FAWM
Sinusitis (Acute)
Elliott Perow, MD
George R. Zlupko, MD, FACEP
Thrush
Paula Diaz, DO
Laura Stone Ellis, MD
Tonsillitis/Pharyngitis
John Rains, MD
Laura Stone Ellis, MD

EYE
Blepharitis
Jonathan Dillen, MD
Ellen Finney, MD
Conjunctivitis
Cameron T. Bubar, DO, MPH
Ellen Finney, MD
Corneal Abrasion
Ankit Patel, MD
Kayla Jester, PA-C
Orbital Cellulitis
Matthew Dillon, MD
Kimberly Fox, MD
Periorbital/Preseptal Cellulitis
Matthew Rizzotti, DO
Kimberly Fox, MD

GASTROINTESTINAL
Appendicitis
Sean Dinallo, MD
Jenna M. Fredette, MD
Cholangitis/Cholecystitis
Hayden J. Schenker, MD
Leila Getto, MD
Clostridioides Difficile Infection
Daniel Doherty, MD
Benjamin Golden, MD
Diverticulitis
Alexander Scott, DO
Stefanie Golebiewski-Manchin, MD

Infectious Diarrhea
Daniel Osarfo-Akoto, MD
Emily Granitto, MD, FACEP
Peritoneal Dialysis-Related Peritonitis
Gregory A. Esparza, MD, PhD
Lisa Kotler, PA-C
Peritonitis/Perforated Viscus/ Intra-abdominal Abscess
Elizabeth Shanahan, MD
Katherine Greco, MD
Spontaneous Bacterial Peritonitis
Taj Shorter, MD
Kathryn Groner, MD, FACEP

GENITOURINARY
Bacterial Vaginosis
Greg A. Esparza, MD, PhD
Kyle Haniszewski, MD
Balanitis
Blythe Fiscella, MD
Michael Hansen II, DO
Endometritis
Brady Stallman, MD
Evan Hawbaker, MD
Epididymitis/Orchitis
Christopher Fong, MD
J. Daniel Hess, MD
Herpes Simplex Virus
Tim Truman, DO
J. Daniel Hess, MD
Pelvic Inflammatory Disease
Sarah Frantz, MD
Robert Hsu, MD
Prostatitis
Prabhdeep Uppal, DO, MS
Robert Hsu, MD
Pyelonephritis
Parth S. Gandhi, DO
Stephen Koczirka, MD
Sexual Assault/STI Prophylaxis
Mary Voelker, DO
Debra Ravert, MD
Syphilis
Joseph Godovchik, MD
Debra Ravert, MD
Trichomoniasis
Alexander Waggener, MD
Debra Ravert, MD
Urethritis/Cervicitis
Stephen Gragg, MD, PhD
Stephen Koczirka, MD
UTI/Cystitis
Diane Y. Wang, MD
Jennifer Empfield, PharmD, BCPS

CONTRIBUTORS

Vulvovaginal Candidiasis
Carine Gregory, MD
Yolanda J. Angstadt, PA-C

PULMONARY
AECB and COPD
Kirsten Ward, MD
Matthew Cruikshank, PA-C
Bronchitis
Amber Higgins, MD
Patrick Matthews, MD
Influenza
Christopher Parronchi, MD
Jonathan McGhee, DO, FACEP
Pneumonia (Adult - Inpatient)
W. Brandon White, DO
Ashling Cook, PharmD
Jason E. Nace, MD
Pneumonia (Pediatric)
Sarah Frantz, MD
Jason E. Nace, MD
Pneumonia (Aspiration with Lung Abscess/Empyema)
Kelly Ware, MD
John T. Powell, MD, MHCDS, FACEP
Tuberculosis
Maria D. Jones, DO
Lori Felker, DHSc, PA-C

SKIN & SOFT TISSUE
Animal/Human Bite Wounds
Jeffrey Watkins, MD
Jeremiah White, MD
Bartholin's Cyst/Abscess
Travis Kaiser Jones, DO
Erin E. Watson, MD, FACEP, CPE
Cellulitis and Abscess
Christian Kasianko, MD
Jonathan Talmud, MD
Diabetic Ulcers
Sarah Wilson, MD
Felon
Sahar Q. Khan, MD
Kristina Stransky, MD
Folliculitis
Sahar Q. Khan, MD
Kristina Stransky, MD
Impetigo
Lynda Yu, MD
Justin C. Stowens, MD, FACEP, RDMS
Mastitis
Lynda Yu, MD
Justin C. Stowens, MD, FACEP, RDMS
Necrotizing Fasciitis
Tim Truman, DO
Timothy Soo, MD

Paronychia
Ryan Lee, MD
Stephen Senichka, DO
Tinea
Douglas Ader, DO
Stephen Senichka, DOD
Varicella or Zoster
Eric Lieu, MD
Robert A. Rosenbaum, MD, FACEP, FAEMS

BIOTERRORISM
Gregory Wanner, DO (all chapters)
Anthrax
Isaac J. Bennett, DO
Botulism
Sanjay Nadesan, MD
Smallpox
Zachariah Brown, DO
Tularemia
Christopher Parronchi, MD
Yersinia
Niketu Patel, MD, MPH

ENVIRONMENTAL EXPOSURES
Rabies
Tulsi D. Patel, MD
Francis Squadrito, MD
Tetanus
Sergiu Costinas, MD
Amit Padaki, MD, MS

IMMUNE-COMPROMISED HOST INFECTIONS
Cryptococcus Neoformans
Paula Diaz, DO
Ross E. Megargel, DO, FACEP, FAEMS
Febrile Neutropenia
Matthew Rizzotti, DO
Jennifer T. Mink, MD
Pneumocystis Jiroveci Pneumonia
Joshua Drake, MD
Michael Morton-Wiedner, MD
Toxoplasmosis
Elizabeth Shanahan, MD
Michael Morton-Wiedner, MD

OCCUPATIONAL POST-EXPOSURE PROPHYLAXIS
HIV and Hepatitis
Greg A. Esparza, MD, PhD
Arayel Osborne, MD

PEDIATRIC INFECTIONS
Johnny Rowles, MD (all)
Lice
Alexander Waggener, MD

Pinworms
Zachariah Brown, DO
Scabies/Mites
Carine Gregory, MD

SEPSIS
Jesse Liou, MD
Christian Coletti, MD, MHCDS

ARTHROPOD-BORNE DISEASE AND PARASITIC INFECTIONS
Babesiosis
Kelly Ware, MD
Eileen DeAngelis, PA-C
Ehrlichiosis/Anaplasmosis
Young Daniel Cho, DO
Michael Diamond, PA-C
Lyme Disease
Daniel Doherty, MD
Danielle DiNorscia, PA-C
Malaria
Matthew Dillon, MD
Robert Donovan, PA-C
Neurocysticercosis
Jessica Beadle, MD
Scott Edmondson, PA-C
Rocky Mountain Spotted Fever
Christopher Fong, MD
Jason Fay, PA-C

APPENDICES
Raymond Sanders, PA-C
Adverse Reactions and Drug Interactions
Frank Mayer, DO, MBA
Michael N. Perza, PharmD, BCPS
Anuj Parikh, MD, FACEP
Cephalosporin Reference
Katherine Ren, DO
Edward Knox, PA-C
Penicillin/Cephalosporin Allergy Algorithm
Hayden J. Schenker, MD
Brent Passarello, MD
Ideal Body Weight Chart
Antibiotic Cost Table
Jonathan Bodner, MD
Eli Zeserson, MD
Pregnancy/Lactation Safety
Parth S. Gandhi, DO
Michael Schuh, PA-C
Antibiotic Coverage Table
Brittney Bunkis, MD
Carolyn Weeks, PA-C
Common Pediatric Dosing
Antibiogram
Dustin Slagle, MD
Jason T. Nomura, MD

TABLE OF CONTENTS

DISCITIS/VERTEBRAL OSTEOMYELITIS

Common organisms: *S. aureus* (most common in U.S.), *Streptococcus* spp., *Pseudomonas* spp., *E. coli* (most common worldwide)
- Vancomycin 25–30 mg/kg IV loading dose **THEN** 15–20 mg/kg IV two-three times daily **PLUS:**
  - Cefepime 2 g IV three times daily **OR**
  - Ciprofloxacin 400 mg IV three times daily
- If vancomycin allergy/intolerance: daptomycin 6-8 mg/kg IV once daily

PEARLS
- Culture of blood, bone, and/or disc is essential to identify causative agent
- Consider withholding empiric antimicrobial therapy until microbiologic diagnosis is confirmed in a stable patient without neurologic deficits
- Risk factors include IV drug use, endocarditis, prior spinal surgery, diabetes, corticosteroid therapy
- Treatment duration generally 6 weeks or longer

INFECTIOUS TENOSYNOVITIS

Common organisms: *S. aureus, Streptococcus* spp., MRSA, gram-negative rods, mixed flora
- Vancomycin 25–30 mg/kg IV loading dose **THEN** 15–20 mg/kg IV two-three times daily **PLUS:**
  - Ceftriaxone 1 g IV once daily (consider 2 g if > 100 kg or severe infection) **OR**
  - Levofloxacin 750 mg IV once daily

Adult Bite Wound

Common organisms: *S. aureus, Streptococcus* spp., *Fusobacterium, Bacteroides* spp., *Pasteurella multocida* (cat), *Eikenella corrodens* (human), *Capnocytophaga canimorsus* (dog)
- Ampicillin/sulbactam 1.5–3 g IV four times daily
- Ceftriaxone 1 g IV once daily (consider 2 g if > 100 kg or severe infection) **AND** metronidazole 500 mg IV three times daily
- If severe PCN allergy:
  - Levofloxacin 750 mg IV once daily **AND** metronidazole 500 mg IV three times daily
- If MRSA suspected:
  - **ADD** vancomycin 15–20 mg/kg IV two-three times daily

2022 EMRA Antibiotic Guide

Ⓟ = Pediatric dosing

Pediatric Bite Wound

Common organisms: *S. aureus*, MRSA, *Pasteurella*
- Ampicillin/sulbactam 50 mg/kg IV four times daily
- Ceftriaxone 100 mg/kg IV once daily **AND** metronidazole 10 mg/kg IV three times daily
- If MRSA suspected:
  - **ADD** vancomycin 15 mg/kg IV four times daily
- If severe PCN allergy:
  - Clindamycin 10 mg/kg IV three times daily **AND** TMP/SMX 5 mg/kg IV two times daily

Disseminated gonococcal infection with chlamydial coverage
- Ceftriaxone 1 g IV once daily (consider 2 g if > 100 kg or severe infection) **PLUS:**
  - Doxycycline 100 mg PO two times daily **OR**
  - Azithromycin 1 g PO once

PEARLS
- Surgical consult required
- Update tetanus immunization if indicated
- If water-related injury, consider additional coverage for mycobacteria or *Pseudomonas* in consultation with ID
- Kanavel's 4 cardinal signs: symmetric swelling of the entire digit ("sausage digit"), held in slight flexion, tenderness along flexor tendon sheath, and pain with passive extension

OPEN FRACTURE

Common organisms: *S. aureus,* coagulase-negative staphylococci, polymicrobial

Open Fracture (based on Gustilo Classification)
- **Type I injury:** open fracture with < 1 cm clean laceration and minimal soft tissue damage
- **Type II injury:** open fracture with 1-10 cm clean laceration without extensive soft tissue injury, flaps, or avulsion
  - Cefazolin 2 g (Ⓟ 30 mg/kg) IV three times daily
  - If severe PCN allergy or MRSA suspected:
    - Vancomycin 15–20 mg/kg IV two–three times daily (Ⓟ 15 mg/kg IV four times daily)

BONE & JOINT

- If injury associated with fresh water exposure, consider *Pseudomonas* coverage
- If injury associated with sea water exposure, consider *Vibrio* coverage
  - Doxycycline 100 mg IV two times daily
- **Type III injury:** open fracture > 10 cm with extensive soft tissue damage including muscle, skin, and neurovascular structures; traumatic amputation; arterial injury that requires repair; or heavily contaminated/farm injury
  - Choose **ONE** antibiotic from Type I/Type II treatment and **ADD** gentamicin 5–7 mg/kg IV once daily (*weight-based dosing*) (Ⓟ 2.5 mg/kg IV three times daily)
  - If concern for *Clostridia* because of soil contamination **ADD:**
    - Penicillin G 5 million units (Ⓟ 25,000 unit/g) IV four times daily **OR**
    - Metronidazole 500 mg (Ⓟ 10 mg/kg) IV three times daily

PEARLS

- Irrigate and administer antibiotics as soon as possible
- Update tetanus immunization if indicated
- Type I and II duration of therapy should not exceed 24 hrs after wound closure. Type III duration should continue for 72 hrs after the injury **OR** antibiotics should be discontinued within 24 hrs after soft tissue closure
- For more information about bone and joint injury, see the EMRA Ortho Guide

OSTEOMYELITIS

Adult: Empiric Regimen

Common organisms: *S. aureus*, coagulase-negative staphylococci, aerobic gram-negative bacilli

- Vancomycin 25–30 mg/kg IV loading dose **THEN** 15–20 mg/kg IV two–three times daily **AND:**
  - Ceftriaxone 2 g IV once daily
  - If *Pseudomonas* spp. suspected (including IV drug use, puncture wound), **REPLACE** ceftriaxone with:
    - Cefepime 2 g IV three times daily **OR**
    - Ciprofloxacin 400 mg IV three times daily

Pediatric: Empiric Regimen

Common organisms: *S. aureus,* Group A *Streptococcus*

- Vancomycin 15 mg/kg IV four times daily
- If *Pseudomonas* spp. suspected (including puncture wound):
  - **ADD** cefepime 50 mg/kg IV three times daily

Ⓟ = Pediatric dosing

Pediatric: Sickle Cell Disease (or incomplete Hib immunization)

Common organisms: *Salmonella, S. aureus*, encapsulated bacteria

- Ceftriaxone 100 mg/kg IV once daily **AND** vancomycin 15 mg/kg IV four times daily

PEARLS

- Consider withholding empiric antimicrobial therapy in a stable patient until cultures obtained
- For hardware involvement, consider consultation with ID
- Ability to probe to bone on exam has high sensitivity and specificity
- X-ray findings lag at least 2 weeks behind clinical infection
  - Normal x-ray does not exclude diagnosis
  - MRI with and without contrast is preferred imaging modality
- Alternative: daptomycin 6–10 mg/kg IV once daily provides satisfactory bone penetration for MRSA coverage

SEPTIC ARTHRITIS

Non-Gonococcal

Common organisms: *S. aureus, Streptococcus* spp., *Pseudomonas* spp., *Enterococcus, B. burgdorferi*

- Vancomycin 25–30 mg/kg IV loading dose **THEN** 15–20 mg/kg IV two–three times daily (Ⓟ 15 mg/kg IV four times daily) **AND** ceftriaxone 1 g (Ⓟ 100 mg/kg) IV once daily (consider 2 g if > 100 kg or severe infection)
  - If *Pseudomonas* spp. suspected (including IV drug use, immunosuppression, or trauma), **REPLACE** ceftriaxone with:
    - Cefepime 2 g (Ⓟ 50 mg/kg) IV three times daily **OR**
    - Ciprofloxacin 400 mg IV three times daily

Gonococcal

- Ceftriaxone 1 g (Ⓟ 100 mg/kg) IV once daily (consider 2 g if > 100 kg or severe infection)

PEARLS

- Surgical consultation for joint washout
- For hardware involvement, consider consultation with ID
- Joint aspirate typically shows WBC > 50,000 with PMN predominance (although up to 1/3 may have less)
- For suspected gonococcal infections
  - Culture blood, urethra, cervix, urine, and joint fluid and consider cultures of throat and rectum
  - Treatment for concurrent *Chlamydia trachomatis* (see p. 47)

SEPTIC BURSITIS

Common organisms: *S. aureus* (> 80%), *Streptococcus* spp., polymicrobial

Mild Inflammation: Outpatient
(Treatment duration 10 days)

- Cephalexin 500 mg PO four times daily **OR** amoxicillin 875 mg PO two times daily **OR** cefuroxime 500 mg PO two times daily **PLUS**:
  - TMP/SMX DS 1–2 tabs PO two times daily **OR**
  - Doxycycline 100 mg PO two times daily
- If severe PCN allergy:
  - Clindamycin 450 mg PO three times daily

Severe Inflammation: Inpatient

- Cefazolin 1–2 g IV three times daily **PLUS**:
  - Vancomycin 25–30 mg/kg IV loading dose **THEN** 15–20 mg/kg IV two–three times daily **OR**
  - Daptomycin 6 mg/kg IV once daily **OR**
  - Linezolid 600 mg IV two times daily

PEARLS

- Diagnosis of septic bursitis should be considered if evidence of pain, swelling, erythema, warmth, fever, or trauma; passive range of motion is usually preserved
- For immunosuppressed patients with traumatic bursitis, **ADD** coverage for *Pseudomonas* spp.
- Severe infections may require repeated drainage

Ⓟ = Pediatric dosing

ENDOCARDITIS

If patient's clinical status allows, obtain cultures first, then promptly administer empiric antibiotics

Native Valve – Acute (days)

Common organisms: *S. aureus*, beta-hemolytic streptococci, *viridans* group streptococci, aerobic gram-negative bacilli
- Vancomycin 25–30 mg/kg IV loading dose **THEN** 15–20 mg/kg IV two–three times daily **AND** ceftriaxone 2 g IV once daily
  - If severe PCN allergy:
    - Ciprofloxacin 400 mg IV two times daily

Native Valve – Subacute (weeks)

Common organisms: *S. aureus*, *viridans* group streptococci, enterococci, *Coxiella burnetii*, and HACEK organisms
- Vancomycin 25–30 mg/kg IV loading dose **THEN** 15–20 mg/kg IV two–three times daily **PLUS:**
  - Ampicillin/sulbactam 3 g IV four times daily **OR**
  - Ceftriaxone 2 g IV once daily
  - If severe PCN allergy:
    - Ciprofloxacin 400 mg IV two times daily

Native Valve – IV Drug Use

Common organism: *S. aureus,* coagulase-negative staphylococci, beta-hemolytic streptococci, aerobic gram-negative bacilli, *Pseudomonas* spp.
- Vancomycin 25–30 mg/kg IV loading dose **THEN** 15–20 mg/kg IV two–three times daily **AND** cefepime 2 g IV three times daily
  - If severe PCN allergy:
    - Ciprofloxacin 400 mg IV two times daily **OR**
    - Aztreonam 2 g IV three times daily

Prosthetic Valve < 1 year post-op

Common organisms: *S. aureus*, coagulase negative staphylococci, aerobic gram-negative bacilli, *Corynebacterium* spp., legionella
- Vancomycin 25–30 mg/kg IV loading dose **THEN** 15–20 mg/kg IV two–three times daily **AND** cefepime 2 g IV three times daily
  - If severe PCN allergy:
    - Ciprofloxacin 400 mg IV two times daily

Prosthetic Valve > 1 year post-op

Common organisms: Staphylococci, *viridans* group streptococci, enterococci

▪ Vancomycin 25–30 mg/kg IV loading dose **THEN** 15–20 mg/kg IV two–three times daily **AND** ceftriaxone 2 g IV once daily

   — If severe PCN allergy:

      • Ciprofloxacin 400 mg IV two times daily

PEARLS

▪ HACEK = Haemophilus spp., *Aggregatibacter* spp., *Cardiobacterium hominis*, *Eikenella corrodens*, and *Kingella* spp.

▪ Some advocate delaying antibiotic initiation until after culture results in patients without acute symptoms or critical illness (eg. sepsis)

▪ IDSA recommends at least 3 sets of blood cultures from **different** venipuncture sites with 1 hour between the first and last sets

▪ TTE should be performed in all cases of suspected infective endocarditis

▪ Rifampin and gentamicin should be withheld pending ID consultant or culture susceptibility results

▪ Implanted devices should not have the pocket sampled

CNS

BELL'S PALSY

Common organisms: *Herpes simplex virus* (HSV), *Herpes Zoster, B. burgdorferi* (Lyme)

PEARLS

- Send Lyme titer in endemic areas, use clinical judgment to treat
- Ensure proper eye protection with artificial tears or ointment to prevent corneal ulceration during recovery
- Without medications more than half of patients recover in 3 months and most patients recover in 9 months
- Imaging not necessary unless there are recurrent or additional neurologic findings, or suspected trauma
- Literature supports an improved rate of recovery with steroids (prednisone 60–80 mg PO daily for 7–10 days) when initiated within 72 hrs of onset (for patients 16 years or older)
- If severe symptoms or high suspicion for HSV, **ADD** antiviral to steroid regimen
  - Acyclovir 400 mg PO five times daily (Ⓟ 20 mg/kg PO four times daily, max 200 mg/dose) for 10 days **OR**
  - Valacyclovir 1 g PO three times daily for 7–10 days

ENCEPHALITIS

Common organisms: HSV, VZV, and CMV

HSV, VZV, or undifferentiated infection

- Acyclovir 10 mg/kg (Ⓟ 10–15 mg/kg) IV three times daily (*dosing based on IBW, consider adjusting if obese*)

Cytomegalovirus

- Ganciclovir 5 mg/kg IV two times daily **AND** foscarnet 90 mg/kg IV two times daily

Ehrlichia/Rickettsia (tick-borne pathogens)

- Doxycycline 200 mg IV once **THEN** 100 mg IV two times daily

PEARLS

- Acyclovir should be initiated in **ALL** patients with suspected encephalitis, pending results of diagnostic studies
- Initiate doxycycline in **ALL** patients with clinical suspicion for tick-borne illness
- Other pathogens include arboviruses (eg, West Nile, equine), EBV, HIV, rabies, and toxoplasmosis

MENINGITIS

Neonate to 1 Month

Common organisms: Group B *Streptococcus* (GBS), *E. coli*, *Listeria* spp., *Klebsiella* spp.

- Ampicillin 50 mg/kg IV four times daily (three times daily < 1 wk old) **AND** gentamicin 2.5 mg/kg IV three times daily (two times daily < 1 wk old) **AND** cefepime 50 mg/kg IV two–three times daily
- If MRSA suspected:
  - **ADD** vancomycin 15 mg/kg IV three times daily (two times daily < 1 wk old)
- Consider coverage for HSV meningoencephalitis with acyclovir 20 mg/kg IV three times daily

1 Month to Adult

Common organisms: *S. pneumoniae, N. meningitidis, H. influenzae,* (GBS and *E. coli* for 1 to 23 months old)

- Vancomycin 25–30 mg/kg IV loading dose **THEN** 15–20 mg/kg IV two–three times daily (Ⓟ 15 mg/kg IV four times daily) **AND** ceftriaxone 2 g (Ⓟ 50 mg/kg) IV two times daily
  - If *Listeria* suspected (> 50 yrs old or immunocompromised):
    - **ADD** ampicillin 2 g IV six times daily (Ⓟ 75 mg/kg IV four times daily)
- If severe PCN allergy:
  - Vancomycin 25–30 mg/kg IV loading dose **THEN** 15–20 mg/kg IV two–three times daily (Ⓟ 15 mg/kg IV four times daily) **PLUS:**
    - Meropenem 2 g (Ⓟ 40 mg/kg) IV three times daily **OR**
    - Ciprofloxacin 400 mg IV three times daily
    - If *Listeria* suspected:
      - **ADD** TMP/SMX 5 mg/kg IV four times daily
- Consider coverage for HSV meningoencephalitis with acyclovir 10 mg/kg (Ⓟ 10–15 mg/kg) IV three times daily (*dosing based on IBW, consider adjusting if obese*)

Cryptococcal Meningitis

- Flucytosine 25 mg/kg PO four times daily **PLUS:**
  - Amphotericin B (liposomal) 4 mg/kg IV once daily **OR**
  - Amphotericin B (lipid complex) 5 mg/kg IV once daily

CNS

Suspected Tuberculosis Meningitis

- Rifampin 600 mg (⊞ 15-20 mg/kg) PO/IV once daily **AND** isoniazid 300 mg (⊞ 10-15 mg/kg) PO once daily **AND**
  - Pyrazinamide dosing per IBW (⊞ 30-40 mg/kg) PO once daily
    - **40-55 kg:** 1 g PO once daily
    - **56-75 kg:** 1.5 g PO once daily
    - **> 75 kg:** 2 g PO once daily

  AND
  - Ethambutol dosing per IBW (⊞ 15-25 mg/kg) PO once daily
    - **40-55 kg:** 800 mg PO once daily
    - **56-75 kg:** 1.2 g PO once daily
    - **> 75 kg:** 1.6 g PO once daily
- Consider initiation of adjunctive corticosteroid therapy with dexamethasone 0.4 mg/kg/day PO/IV once daily OR prednisolone 2-4 mg/kg/day (max 40 mg) PO once daily

Post-neurosurgery, penetrating head trauma, CSF shunt

Common organisms: gram-negative rods (including *P. aeruginosa*), *Staph* spp., *P. acnes* (CSF shunt)

- Vancomycin 15–20 mg/kg IV two–three times daily (⊞ 15 mg/kg IV four times daily) **PLUS:**
  - Cefepime 2 g (⊞ 50 mg/kg) IV three times daily **OR**
  - Meropenem 2 g (⊞ 40 mg/kg) IV three times daily

Prophylaxis for *N. meningitidis* (not recommended for other organisms)

For all household contacts, childcare contacts, or DIRECT exposure to patient's oral secretions (kissing, mouth-to-mouth resuscitation, endotracheal intubation/ management) occurring within 7 days prior to patient presentation

- Ceftriaxone 250 mg (⊞ < 15 years old, 125 mg) IM once
- Ciprofloxacin 500 mg PO once (⊞ not recommended if < 18 years old or pregnant/breastfeeding)
- Rifampin 600 mg (⊞ < 1 month old, 5 mg/kg; ≥ 1 month old, 10 mg/kg) PO two times daily for 2 days

PEARLS

- Do not delay antibiotic therapy for LP or imaging
- Indications for obtaining CT prior to LP
  - Immunocompromised, history of CNS disease (mass lesion, stroke, or infection), new onset seizure, papilledema, abnormal level of consciousness, focal neurological deficit
- For suspected pneumococcal meningitis (all patients) or *H. influenzae* (pediatrics), **ADD** dexamethasone 0.15 mg/kg IV four times daily **before or in conjunction** with the first dose of antibiotics

SPINAL OR INTRACRANIAL EPIDURAL ABSCESS

Common organisms: *Staphylococcus* spp., *Streptococcus* spp., gram-negative bacilli

- Vancomycin 25-30 mg/kg IV loading dose **THEN** 15-20 mg/kg IV two-three times daily (ⓟ 15 mg/kg IV four times daily) **AND** ceftriaxone 2 g (ⓟ 50 mg/kg) IV once daily
- If *Pseudomonas* suspected, **REPLACE** ceftriaxone with:
  - Cefepime 2 g (ⓟ 50 mg/kg) IV three times daily
- If severe PCN allergy **CONSIDER REPLACING** ceftriaxone with meropenem 2 g (ⓟ 40 mg/kg) IV three times daily

PEARLS

- Classic triad of back pain, fever, and neurologic deficit is present in only 10-15% of patients
- Suspect *Pseudomonas* in penetrating trauma, recent neurosurgery, CSF shunt, immunocompromised patients, IVDU
- Consider fungal, toxoplasmosis, or tuberculous infections in immunocompromised patients
- In stable patients, consider delaying antibiotic treatment until abscess fluid obtained for culture
- MRI with and without contrast is the test of choice

EAR/NOSE/THROAT

ACUTE NECROTIZING ULCERATIVE GINGIVITIS (ANUG)

Common organisms: *Fusobacterium, Treponema, Prevotella, Bacteroides* spp.
(Treatment duration: 7–10 days)
- Metronidazole 500 mg PO three times daily
- Amoxicillin/clavulanate 875 mg PO two times daily
- If HIV positive, consider **ADDING:**
  - Nystatin rinses 5 mL four times daily for 7–14 days **OR**
  - Fluconazole 200 mg PO daily for 7–14 days

PEARLS

- Diagnostic triad includes pain, ulcerated interdental papillae, and gingival bleeding; may include gingival edema, gray pseudomembranes over ulcerations, and halitosis
- Gentle debridement with gauze or cotton swab is recommended to remove pseudomembrane and debris
- Pain control with topical viscous 2% lidocaine 15 mL PO every 6 hrs (rinse and spit), ibuprofen
- Saline rinses can help to speed resolution; oral rinses with a hydrogen peroxide 3% solution or chlorhexidine 0.12% two times daily during treatment may be of benefit
- May progress to Vincent angina (tonsillar, pharyngeal involvement): searing pharyngeal pain, fever, and regional lymphadenopathy

DENTAL ABSCESS

Common organisms: Polymicrobial oral flora
(Treatment duration: 7–14 days)
- Penicillin VK 500 mg PO four times daily
- Amoxicillin/clavulanate 875 mg PO two times daily
- Clindamycin 450 mg PO three times daily or 600 mg IV three times daily
- Ampicillin/sulbactam 3 g IV four times daily

EPIGLOTTITIS

Common organisms: Group A *Streptococcus, H. parainfluenzae, S. pneumoniae, S. aureus, H. influenzae*
- Ceftriaxone 1 g (P 50 mg/kg) IV once daily (consider 2 g if > 100 kg or severe infection)

- Ampicillin/sulbactam 3 g (⊕ 50 mg/kg) IV four times daily
- If severe PCN allergy: **CONSIDER** levofloxacin 750 mg IV once daily

Severe Infection or Immunocompromised

Common organisms: As above, **PLUS** *C. albicans, Pseudomonas* spp.

- Cefepime 2 g (⊕ 50 mg/kg) IV three times daily **AND** vancomycin 25-30 mg/kg IV loading dose, **THEN** 15–20 mg/kg IV two–three times daily (⊕ 15 mg/kg IV four times daily)

PEARLS

- Close airway monitoring is warranted
- Use of steroids and racemic epinephrine is controversial
- Consider adding antifungal agent in consultation with ID for immunocompromised patients

LUDWIG'S ANGINA

Common organisms: Polymicrobial oral flora

- Ampicillin/sulbactam 3 g (⊕ 50 mg/kg) IV four times daily
- Ceftriaxone 2 g (⊕ 100 mg/kg) IV once daily **AND** metronidazole 500 mg IV two times daily (⊕ 10 mg/kg IV three times daily)
- If severe PCN allergy:
  - Clindamycin 600 mg (⊕ 10 mg/kg) IV three times daily **AND** levofloxacin 750 mg (⊕ 10 mg/kg) IV once daily

Immunocompromised

Common organisms: As above, **PLUS** *Pseudomonas* spp.

- Piperacillin/tazobactam 4.5 g (⊕ 80 mg/kg) IV four times daily
- Cefepime 2 g (⊕ 50 mg/kg) IV three times daily **AND** metronidazole 500 mg (⊕ 10 mg/kg) IV three times daily
- Imipenem 1 g IV three times daily (⊕ 20 mg/kg IV four times daily)
- If MRSA suspected:
  - **ADD** vancomycin 25-30 mg/kg IV loading dose, **THEN** 15–20 mg/kg IV two–three times daily to any of the above regimens

PEARLS

- Clinical findings: "hot potato" voice, dysphagia, drooling, stridor, trismus, tongue elevation, edema of the floor of mouth, high fever
- Consider early surgical consultation
- Consider adding antifungal agent in consultation with ID

MASTOIDITIS

Common organisms: *S. pneumoniae, S. pyogenes, S. aureus*/MRSA, *H. influenzae, P. aeruginosa, M. catarrhalis*

- Vancomycin 25–30 mg/kg IV loading dose **THEN** 15–20 mg/kg IV two–three times daily (P 15 mg/kg IV four times daily) **AND** ceftriaxone 2 g (P 100 mg/kg) IV once daily
- If *Pseudomonas* suspected (chronic otitis or previous ABx use):
  - Cefepime 2 g (P 50 mg/kg) IV three times daily **OR**
  - Piperacillin/tazobactam 4.5 g (P 80 mg/kg) IV four times daily
- If severe PCN allergy:
  - Aztreonam 2 g IV three times daily (P 30 mg/kg IV four times daily)

PEARLS

- Presents as acute otitis media **PLUS** postauricular edema, erythema, tenderness, fluctuance, or displacement of the auricle/pinna
- Consider CT or MRI of temporal bones and intracranial cavity to exclude osteomyelitis, cholesteatoma, or abscess
- Consider ENT consultation

OTITIS EXTERNA

Acute Otitis Externa (swimmer's ear)

Common organisms: *P. aeruginosa, Staphylococcus* spp., *Peptostreptococcus* spp., *Bacteroides* spp.
(Treatment duration: 7–10 days)

- Polymyxin B/neomycin/hydrocortisone 4 drops (P 3 drops) four times daily (avoid if TM perforated)
- Ofloxacin 0.3% otic solution 10 drops (P 5 drops) once daily
- Ciprofloxacin/hydrocortisone 3 drops (P 3 drops) two times daily
- Ciprofloxacin/dexamethasone 4 drops (P 4 drops) two times daily
- Acetic acid 2.0%/hydrocortisone otic 5 drops (P 5 drops) four times daily
- Ciprofloxacin 500 mg PO two times daily (for severe acute otitis externa extending outside the ear canal or immunocompromised patient)

PEARLS

- Consider cerumen removal to expedite resolution
- Insert wick to administer drops for 48 hrs if external ear canal is edematous
- 2021: "You're on mute."

Malignant Otitis Externa

Common organisms: *P. aeruginosa*
- Ciprofloxacin 400 mg IV three times daily (Ⓟ 10 mg/kg IV two times daily)
- Piperacillin/tazobactam 4.5 g (Ⓟ 60 mg/kg) IV four times daily
- Cefepime 2 g (Ⓟ 50 mg/kg) IV three times daily
- Meropenem 2 g (Ⓟ 20 mg/kg) IV three times daily

PEARLS
- For immunocomprised or diabetic patients, consider antifungals
- CT or MRI scan may be utilized to determine extent of disease

OTITIS MEDIA

Common organisms: *S. pneumoniae, H. influenzae, M. catarrhalis, S. pyogenes, S. aureus,* respiratory viruses
(Treatment duration: 5–7 days unless otherwise noted)

No antibiotics in prior month
- Amoxicillin 875 mg (Ⓟ 45 mg/kg) PO two times daily
  - Treatment duration: 5-7 days if ≥ 2 yrs old; 10 days if < 2 yrs old or with acute TM perforation

Antibiotics in prior month
- Amoxicillin/clavulanate 45 mg/kg PO two times daily
- Cefuroxime 15 mg/kg PO two times daily
- Cefdinir 14 mg/kg PO once daily
- Cefpodoxime 5 mg/kg PO two times daily
- Ceftriaxone 50 mg/kg IM once daily for 3 days

Treatment failure (no change in ear pain, fever, bulging TM, otorrhea after 3 days treatment)
- Amoxicillin/clavulanate 45 mg/kg PO two times daily for 10 days
- Ceftriaxone 50 mg/kg IM once daily for 3 days

Severe PCN allergy
- Consider third-generation cephalosporin (*see Penicillin/Cephalosporin Allergy Algorithm, p. 102*)
- Clindamycin 10 mg/kg PO three times daily (does not cover *H. influenzae* or *M. catarrhalis*) **OR**
- Azithromycin 10 mg/kg PO once, **THEN** 5 mg/kg PO once daily for 4 days (limited efficacy against *H. influenzae* and *S. pneumoniae*)

PEARLS

- Consider "wait and see" approach for 48–72 hrs in non-severe, unilateral AOM in children > 6 months
- Recommend antibiotics for infants < 6 months, bilateral ear involvement, otorrhea, severe symptoms (otalgia > 48 hrs, temp > 39°C)
- Persistent middle ear effusion is common after the resolution of acute symptoms
- Duration of therapy is variable depending on patient age, associated clinical features, and chosen antibiotic

PARAPHARYNGEAL ABSCESS (PERITONSILLAR AND RETROPHARYNGEAL)

Common organisms: *Streptococcus* spp., anaerobes, *Fusobacterium necrophorum, Eikenella corrodens, H. influenzae, S. aureus*

Outpatient
(Treatment duration: 10–14 days)

- Amoxicillin/clavulanate 875 mg (🄿 45 mg/kg) PO two times daily
- Clindamycin 450 mg (🄿 10 mg/kg) PO three times daily

Inpatient

- Ampicillin/sulbactam 3 g (🄿 50 mg/kg) IV four times daily
- Clindamycin 600 mg IV three times daily (🄿 10 mg/kg IV four times daily) **AND** levofloxacin 750 mg (🄿 10 mg/kg) IV once daily
- Metronidazole 500 mg (🄿 10 mg/kg) IV three times daily **PLUS:**
  - Penicillin G 4 million units (🄿 50,000 units/kg) IV four times daily **OR**
  - Ceftriaxone 2 g (🄿 100 mg/kg) IV once daily
- If severe infection or MRSA suspected:
  - **ADD** vancomycin 25-30 mg/kg IV loading dose, **THEN** 15–20 mg/kg IV two three times daily (🄿 15 mg/kg IV four times daily)

PEARLS

- I&D is the treatment of choice
- Consider one-time high dose steroid (dexamethasone 10 mg PO/IV once) for symptomatic relief (limited data in pediatric patients)

PAROTITIS/SIALADENITIS

Common organisms: *S. aureus,* oral flora, mumps (paramyxovirus), enteroviruses, influenza virus

Less common: TB, HIV

Oral Treatment
(Treatment duration: 10–14 days)
- Amoxicillin/clavulanate 875 mg (⊕ 45 mg/kg) PO two times daily
- Clindamycin 450 mg (⊕ 10 mg/kg) PO three times daily
- Cephalexin 500 mg (⊕ 12.5 mg/kg) PO four times daily **AND** metronidazole 500 mg (⊕ 10 mg/kg) PO three times daily

Intravenous Treatment
- Ampicillin/sulbactam 3 g (⊕ 50 mg/kg) IV four times daily
- Metronidazole 500 mg (⊕ 10 mg/kg) IV three times daily **PLUS:**
  - Oxacillin 1 g (⊕ 25 mg/kg) IV four times daily **OR**
  - Cefazolin 1 g (⊕ 30 mg/kg) IV three times daily **OR**
  - Ceftriaxone 1 g (⊕ 50 mg/kg) IV once daily (consider 2 g if > 100 kg or severe infection)
- If MRSA suspected or immunocompromised:
  - **ADD** vancomycin 15–20 mg/kg IV two–three times daily (⊕ 15 mg/kg IV four times daily)

PEARLS
- For simple sialadenitis, consider establishing duct patency with massage, hydration, or stimulation of salivary glands with sialogogues (lemon drops, sour candy, or orange juice)
- Parotid gland stones/tumors and mucous plugs may lead to obstruction and secondary infection, potentially requiring surgical resection
- Dehydration, intubation, anticholinergics, diuretics, TCAs, phenothiazines, and beta-blocker medications are risk factors for bacterial parotitis

PERTUSSIS

Common organism: *Bordetella* spp.

Active Disease/Post-Exposure Prophylaxis
Age < 2 months

- Azithromycin 10 mg/kg PO once daily for 5 days

Age 2-5 months

- Azithromycin 10 mg/kg PO once daily for 5 days
- TMP/SMX (DS) 4 mg/kg PO two times daily for 14 days

Age ≥ 6 months

- Azithromycin 10 mg/kg (max 500 mg/dose) PO once, **THEN** 5 mg/kg (max 250 mg/dose) PO once daily for 4 days
- TMP/SMX (DS) 4 mg/kg (max 160 mg/dose) PO two times daily for 14 days

Adult

- Azithromycin 500 mg PO once, **THEN** 250 mg PO once daily for 4 days
- TMP/SMX (DS) 1 tablet PO two times daily for 14 days

PEARLS

- Timing:
  - Treat patients < 1 year of age and pregnant women within 6 weeks of cough onset
  - Treat patients > 1 year of age within 3 weeks of cough onset
- Consider in any patient with prolonged cough, coughing paroxysms, whoops, or post-tussive emesis
- Post exposure prophylaxis recommended within 21 days for close contacts, especially infants, patients with chronic lung disease, and immunodeficiency
- Pertussis is a clinical diagnosis but can be confirmed through nasopharyngeal culture (gold standard) or PCR
- Extremely contagious (via respiratory droplet) in non-immunized children and adults (> 80% of susceptible individuals exposed will develop the illness)
- Average incubation period is 7–10 days, most infectious in catarrhal stage or the first 3 weeks of cough symptoms
- Most individuals appear to clear infection without antibiotic treatment within 6 weeks
- Immunity wanes 5–10 years after immunization; CDC recommends Tdap for nonpregnant adults and with each pregnancy

EAR/NOSE/THROAT

SINUSITIS (ACUTE)

Common organisms: Viral, *S. pneumoniae, H. influenzae, M. catarrhalis*

 Avoid prescribing antibiotics in the ED for uncomplicated sinusitis

Mild to Moderate Disease
(Treatment duration - adults: 5-7 days)
(Treatment duration - pediatrics: 10-14 days)
- Amoxicillin/clavulanate 875 mg ((P) 22.5 mg/kg) PO two times daily
- If severe PCN allergy:
  - Doxycycline 100 mg PO two times daily **OR**
  - Levofloxacin 750 mg PO once daily

Risk for Resistance or Antibiotic Failure (outpatient)
(Treatment duration: 7-10 days)
- Amoxicillin/clavulanate 2 g PO two times daily ((P) 45 mg/kg PO two times daily for 14 days)
- Levofloxacin 750 mg PO once daily
- Moxifloxacin 400 mg PO once daily

Severe Disease (inpatient)
- Ampicillin/sulbactam 3 g ((P) 50 mg/kg) IV four times daily
- Ceftriaxone 1-2 g IV once daily ((P) 25 mg/kg IV two times daily)
- Levofloxacin 750 mg IV once daily
- Moxifloxacin 400 mg IV once daily

PEARLS
- Majority of cases are viral and will not require antibiotic treatment
- Symptomatic treatment: analgesics, antipyretics, intranasal saline irrigation, and intranasal corticosteroids
- Oral or intranasal decongestants should be avoided in suspected bacterial sinusitis as there is no evidence of efficacy and there is risk of side effects
- Indications for antibiotics
  - No symptom improvement after 10 days
  - Onset with high fever ≥ 39°C and purulent nasal discharge or facial pain ≥ 3-4 days
  - Worsening symptoms following viral URI > 5-6 days that was initially improving
- Imaging is not initially recommended
- Risk for resistance: living in a region with high rates (10%) of penicillin resistant *S. pneumoniae*, recent hospitalization, antibiotic use within past month, or immunocompromised

THRUSH

Common organism: *Candida* spp.

Mild Disease (Adult)
(Treatment duration: 7–14 days)
- Nystatin oral suspension (100,000 units/mL) 5 mL PO four times daily (swish for several minutes and swallow)
- Clotrimazole troches 10 mg PO five times daily (dissolve over 20 min)

Moderate to Severe Disease (Adult)
(Treatment duration: 7–14 days)
- Fluconazole 200 mg PO once, **THEN** 100 mg PO once daily

Refractory Disease
(Treatment duration: up to 28 days)
- Itraconazole oral solution 200 mg PO once daily without food
- Posaconazole suspension 400 mg PO two times daily for 3 days, **THEN** 400 mg PO daily
- Voriconazole 200 mg PO two times daily

Pediatric Dosing
(Treatment duration: 7–14 days)
- Nystatin oral suspension (100,000 units/mL)
  - Infants < 30 days old: 1 mL (0.5 mL to each side of mouth) four times daily
    > 30 days old: 2 mL (1 mL to each side of mouth) four times daily
  - Children: 5 mL PO four times daily (swish and swallow)
- Clotrimazole troches (🅟 choking hazard; use only if > 4 years old) 10 mg (1 lozenge) PO five times daily (dissolve over 20 min)
- Fluconazole: moderate to severe disease in children > 1 yr: 6 mg/kg PO once (max 600 mg/dose), **THEN** 3 mg/kg PO once daily for 13 days (max 200 mg/dose)

PEARLS
- Key difference between thrush and leukoplakia is ability to scrape off thrush
- Thrush usually resolves within 3–4 days of treatment. Discontinue treatment 2 days after lesions disappear
- Treat dentures to prevent recurrences (brush dentures and soak in chlorhexidine gluconate solution nightly)
- Avoid feeding infants and children for 5-10 min after nystatin use
- If bottle feeding, sterilize nipple prior to feeding
- If breastfeeding, mothers must treat their nipples after each feeding
- Additional option for adult mild thrush: miconazole mucoadhesive buccal 50 mg tablet applied to mucosal surface over canine fossa (may be cost-prohibitive)

TONSILLITIS/PHARYNGITIS

Common organisms: Viruses (*mononucleosis, adenovirus, coxsackievirus, HIV, HSV*), Group A beta-hemolytic strep (GABHS), *N. gonorrhea, C. diphtheriae*
Note: The majority of pharyngitis is viral

Adult
(Treatment duration: 10 days unless otherwise noted)
- Benzathine penicillin G 1.2 million units IM once
- Penicillin VK 500 mg PO two times daily
- Amoxicillin 500 mg PO two times daily **OR** 1 g PO once daily
- Cephalexin 500 mg PO two times daily
- Azithromycin 500 mg PO once daily for 5 days
- If severe PCN allergy:
  - Clindamycin 300 mg PO three times daily

Pediatric
(Treatment duration: 10 days unless otherwise noted)
- Benzathine penicillin G < 27 kg 600,000 units IM once; ≥ 27 kg 1.2 million units IM once
- Penicillin VK < 27 kg 250 mg PO two or three times daily; ≥ 27 kg 500 mg PO two times daily
- Amoxicillin 25 mg/kg PO two times daily **OR** 50 mg/kg PO once daily
- Cephalexin 20 mg/kg PO two times daily
- Azithromycin 12 mg/kg PO once daily for 5 days
- Clindamycin 10 mg/kg PO three times daily (max 300 mg/dose)

PEARLS
- GABHS leads to 5–15% of sore throat visits in adults, 20–30% in pediatrics
- Modified Centor criteria (≥ 3 years old) often used to decrease unnecessary ABx
- Symptomatic treatment: topical anesthetics, steroids (dexamethasone 0.6 mg/kg PO once, max 10 mg), and acetaminophen or ibuprofen (IDSA recommends *against* use of steroids in GABHS)
- For suspected mononucleosis, consider heterophile antibody test (sensitivity increases with duration of symptoms); treatment is supportive with steroids, hydration, no contact sports for 6–8 weeks
- For severe pharyngitis, consider gonorrhea treatment; test-of-cure recommended

Modified Centor Criteria ≥ 3 years old	
Tonsillar exudate	+1
Fever/Hx fever > 38°C	+1
Tender anterior cervical lymphadenopathy	+1
Absence of cough	+1
Age 3-14 years	+1
Age 15-44 years	0
Age ≥ 45 years	-1

1 point: ABx generally not indicated
2-3 points: Consider rapid antigen detection testing or throat culture if feasible
4-5 points: Consider ABx treatment

EAR/NOSE/THROAT

BLEPHARITIS

Common organisms: *S. aureus*, coagulase-negative staphylococci, *P. acnes*
Note: Antibiotics are usually not necessary unless local care is unsuccessful.
There are various antibiotic ointment options. Apply to lid margin, up to four
times daily for up to 1 month
- Bacitracin ophthalmic ointment
- Erythromycin ophthalmic ointment

PEARLS

- Hygiene: apply warm compresses to closed lid for 5–10 min 2-4 times daily
  to loosen crusts, **THEN** wash/massage lids with a cotton swab soaked in a
  mixture of baby shampoo and water (1:1 mix)
- Consider artificial tears to treat dry eye
- Treatment of chronic disease may require Ophthalmology follow-up

CONJUNCTIVITIS

Common organisms: Viral, *S. aureus*, *S. pneumoniae*, *H. influenzae*,
M. catarrhalis, *Pseudomonas* spp., *N. gonorrhea*, *C. trachomatis*

Bacterial Conjunctivitis (non-gonococcal, non-chlamydial)
- Erythromycin 0.5% ophthalmic ointment ½ inch (1.25 cm) 4–6 times daily
  for 5–7 days
- Polymyxin B/Trimethoprim sol. 1 drop every 3 hrs while awake for 7–10 days
- Bacitracin/Polymyxin B ophthalmic ointment ½ inch every 3–4 hrs
  for 7–10 days
- Sulfacetamide 10% ophthalmic sol. 1–2 drops every 2–3 hrs for 5–7 days
- Ofloxacin 0.3% 1-2 drops every 2-4 hrs while awake for 2 days, **THEN** 4
  times daily for 5 days
- Ciprofloxacin 0.3% 1-2 drops every 2 hrs while awake for 2 days, **THEN** 4
  times daily for 5 days
- Levofloxacin 0.5% sol. 1–2 drops every 2 hrs while awake for 2 days, **THEN**
  4 times daily for 5 days
- Moxifloxacin 0.5% sol. 1 drop every 8 hrs while awake for 7 days

Suspected Gonococcal/Chlamydial Conjunctivitis - topical above PLUS:
- Ceftriaxone 1 g (ⓟ 50 mg/kg) IM/IV once (consider 2 g if > 100 kg or severe
  infection) **PLUS:**
  - Doxycycline 100 mg PO two times daily for 7 days **OR**
  - Azithromycin 1 g (ⓟ 20 mg/kg) PO once

PEARLS

- Majority of conjunctival infections are viral and do not require treatment
- Sulfacetamide is available, but not first-line therapy due to the possibility of a rare but severe allergic reaction
- Eye drops preferred for adults and ointments preferred for children
- Treat contact lens wearers with fluoroquinolone to cover *Pseudomonas* spp. and counsel to discontinue contact lens use until infection has cleared. Discard lens case, eye drops, and disposable lenses
- Neonatal conjunctivitis: recommend consultation with ID or Neonatology

CORNEAL ABRASION

Note: If corneal ulcer present, more aggressive treatment is required. Recommend consultation with Ophthalmology

Non-Contact Lens User (Treatment duration: 3–5 days)

Common organisms: *Staphylococcus* spp., *Streptococcus* spp.

- Erythromycin 0.5% ophthalmic ointment: ½ inch (1.25 cm) ribbon, apply four times daily
- Sulfacetamide 10% ophthalmic ointment: ½ inch (1.25 cm) ribbon, apply four times daily
- Sulfacetamide 10% sol. 2 drops four times daily
- Ciprofloxacin 0.3% sol. 2 drops four times daily
- Ofloxacin 0.3% sol. 2 drops four times daily

Contact Lens User (Treatment duration: 5 days)

Common organisms: *Pseudomonas* spp.

- Ciprofloxacin 0.3% sol. 2 drops four times daily
- Ofloxacin 0.3% sol. 2 drops four times daily
- Gentamicin 0.3% ophthalmic ointment: ½ inch (1.25 cm) ribbon, three times daily
- Gentamicin 0.3% sol. 2 drops six times daily
- Tobramycin 0.3% sol. 2 drops four times daily

PEARLS

- Eye drops preferred for adults and ointments preferred for children
- In recurrent abrasion, ointment is preferred method of treatment
- Untreated corneal abrasions can progress to corneal ulcers
- Discontinue contact lens use and have 24-hr follow-up with Ophthalmology
- Topical corticosteroids and eye patches are not recommended
- Update tetanus immunization if indicated
- For pain control, consider ophthalmic NSAIDs

EYE

ORBITAL CELLULITIS

Common organisms: *Streptococcus* spp., *Staphylococcus* spp.,
H. influenzae, anaerobes

- Vancomycin 25–30 mg/kg IV loading dose **THEN** 15–20 mg/kg IV two–three times daily (ⓟ 15 mg/kg IV four times daily) **PLUS:**
  - Ampicillin/sulbactam 3 g (ⓟ 50 mg/kg) IV four times daily **OR**
  - Ceftriaxone 2 g (ⓟ 100 mg/kg) IV once daily
  - If severe PCN allergy:
    - Levofloxacin 750 mg (ⓟ 10 mg/kg) PO/IV once daily (≥ 5 yrs); two times daily ages 6 months to 5 yrs (max 750 mg/day)

PEARLS

- Common presentation: pain with eye movement, proptosis, visual changes
- CT scan of orbits/sinuses with contrast may help differentiate from preseptal cellulitis
- Consider MRI/MRV or CT venography to detect cavernous sinus thrombosis
- If odontogenic disease suspected, ensure adequate anaerobic coverage
  - Metronidazole 500 mg IV three-four times daily (if not using ampicillin/sulbactam)
- Consider fungal etiologies (mucormycosis and aspergillus) in refractory cases or patients with immunodeficiency

PERIORBITAL/PRESEPTAL CELLULITIS

Common organisms: *Staphylococcus* spp., *Streptococcus* spp., anaerobes

Outpatient (Treatment duration: 5–7 days)

- Clindamycin 300 mg PO three times daily (ⓟ 10 mg/kg PO four times daily) **OR** TMP/SMX (DS) 1-2 tablets (ⓟ 5 mg/kg) PO two times daily **PLUS:**
  - Amoxicillin/clavulanate 875 mg (ⓟ 45 mg/kg) PO two times daily **OR**
  - Cefdinir 300 mg (ⓟ 7 mg/kg) PO two times daily

Inpatient

- Treat according to orbital cellulitis guidelines

PEARLS

- Close follow-up is strongly recommended
- Indications for CT scan of orbits/sinuses with IV contrast include inability to assess vision secondary to edema, bilateral periorbital edema, proptosis, ophthalmoplegia, change in visual acuity, and no improvement after 24 hrs of outpatient therapy
- Consider admission for patients < 2 yrs old or those with significant comorbidities

APPENDICITIS

Common organisms: *E. coli, Peptostreptococcus, Klebsiella* spp., *Proteus* spp., *Bacteroides* spp.

Simple Appendicitis, Pediatric
- Ceftriaxone 50 mg/kg IV once daily **AND** metronidazole 10 mg/kg IV three times daily
- Ertapenem 15 mg/kg IV two times daily (max 1 g/day)
- Gentamicin 2.5 mg/kg IV three times daily **AND** metronidazole 10 mg/kg IV three times daily
- If severe PCN allergy:
  — Ciprofloxacin 10-15 mg/kg/dose IV two times daily (max 400 mg/dose) **AND** metronidazole 10 mg/kg IV three times daily

Simple Appendicitis, Adult
- Metronidazole 500 mg IV three times daily **PLUS:**
  — Ceftriaxone 1 g IV once daily (consider 2 g if > 100 kg or severe infection) **OR**
  — Levofloxacin 750 mg IV once daily
- Ertapenem 1 g IV once daily

Complicated Appendicitis, Adult and Pediatric
(gangrenous, perforated, abscess, or phlegmon)
- Piperacillin/tazobactam 4.5 g (Ⓟ 80 mg/kg/dose; max 16 g/day) IV three times daily
- Imipenem/cilastatin 1 g (Ⓟ 25 mg/kg) IV three times daily
- Metronidazole 500 mg (Ⓟ 10 mg/kg) IV three times daily **PLUS:**
  — Cefepime 2 g (Ⓟ 50 mg/kg) IV two times daily **OR**
  — Ciprofloxacin 400 mg IV two times daily **OR**
  — Levofloxacin 750 mg IV once daily

PEARLS
- Indications for complicated appendicitis treatment regimen include:
  — Immunocompromised state
  — Poor nutritional status/low albumin level
  — Significant cardiovascular disease/multiple comorbidities
  — Health care associated infections (eg, recent hospitalization, antibiotics, extended care facility residents, etc.)
- The 2020s began with a fair number of karens (not to be confused with Karens)

CHOLANGITIS/CHOLECYSTITIS

Common organisms: *E. Coli, Klebsiella* spp., *Pseudomonas* spp., *Enterobacter* spp., *Enterococcus* spp., *Bacteroides* spp., *Streptococcus* spp., *Staphylococcus* spp.

Mild to Moderate Disease

- ■ Ceftriaxone 1 g IV once daily (consider 2 g if > 100 kg or severe infection)
- ■ Cefazolin 2 g IV three times daily
- ■ If severe PCN allergy:
  - — Levofloxacin 750 mg IV once daily

Severe/Life-Threatening Disease

- ■ Metronidazole 500 mg IV three times daily **PLUS:**
  - — Ceftriaxone 2 g IV once daily (community-acquired) **OR**
  - — Cefepime 2 g IV three times daily
  - — If severe PCN allergy:
    - • Levofloxacin 750 mg IV once daily
- ■ Piperacillin/tazobactam 4.5 g IV four times daily
- ■ Imipenem/cilastatin 1 g IV three times daily
- ■ If MRSA suspected:
  - — **ADD** vancomycin 25–30 mg/kg IV loading dose **THEN** 15–20 mg/kg IV two–three times daily

PEARLS

- ■ Indications for severe/life-threatening treatment regimen
  - — Clinical instability
  - — Health care-associated infections (eg, post-operative)
  - — Recent cephalosporin exposure
  - — Immunocompromised patients
- ■ Indications for MRSA coverage
  - — Known colonization
  - — Prior treatment failure and significant antibiotic exposure
  - — Health care-associated infections
- ■ Empiric therapy not recommended for pancreatitis/necrotizing pancreatitis

CLOSTRIDIOIDES DIFFICILE INFECTIONS (C. DIFF)

(Treatment duration: 10 days)

Initial Episode, Mild-Moderate Disease (WBC < 15,000 cells/mL **OR** serum creatinine level < 1.5 times the premorbid level)
- Fidaxomicin 200 mg PO two times daily
- Vancomycin 125 mg PO four times daily
- Metronidazole 500 mg PO three times daily (only if above agents unavailable)

Initial Episode, Severe Disease (WBC > 15,000 cells/mL **OR** serum creatinine level > 1.5 times the premorbid level)
- Fidaxomicin 200 mg PO two times daily
- Vancomycin 125 mg PO four times daily

Initial Episode, Fulminant (hypotension, shock, ileus, megacolon)
- Metronidazole 500 mg IV three times daily **AND** vancomycin 500 mg PO four times daily
- For ileus, consider adding vancomycin 500 mg in 100 mL saline four times daily as retention enema

PEARLS
- Avoid medications that decrease intestinal motility
- Consider cost of outpatient therapy
- Recommend consultation with ID for cases of recurrence, severe complicated disease, or concurrent antibiotic use

DIVERTICULITIS

Common organisms: *Enterobacteriaceae, Bacteroides* spp., *Enterococcus* spp.

Outpatient Therapy (Treatment duration: 7–10 days)
- Amoxicillin-clavulanate 875 mg PO two times daily
- Metronidazole 500 mg PO three times daily **PLUS:**
  - Ciprofloxacin 500 mg PO two times daily **OR**
  - Levofloxacin 750 mg PO once daily
- Moxifloxacin 400 mg PO once daily

Inpatient Therapy, Mild to Moderate Disease
- Metronidazole 500 mg IV three times daily **PLUS:**
  - Ceftriaxone 1 g IV once daily (consider 2 g if > 100 kg) **OR**
  - Ciprofloxacin 400 mg IV two times daily **OR**
  - Levofloxacin 750 mg IV once daily

GI

- Ertapenem 1 g IV once daily
- Moxifloxacin 400 mg IV once daily

Inpatient Therapy, Severe Disease

- Piperacillin/tazobactam 4.5 g IV three times daily
- Vancomycin 15–20 mg/kg IV two–three times daily **AND** metronidazole 500 mg IV three times daily **PLUS:**
  - Cefepime 1 g IV three times daily **OR**
  - Ciprofloxacin 400 mg IV two times daily **OR**
  - Levofloxacin 750 mg IV once daily
- Imipenem/cilastatin 1 g IV three times daily
- Meropenem 1 g IV three times daily

PEARLS

- Indications for severe disease treatment regimen
  - Health care-associated infections (eg, post-operative)
  - Previous *Enterococcus* treatment
  - Immunocompromised patients
  - Valvular heart disease or intravascular devices
- Indications for MRSA coverage
  - Known colonization
  - Prior treatment failure and significant antibiotic exposure

INFECTIOUS DIARRHEA

Bacteria: *Campylobacter jejuni, C. difficile, E. coli, L. monocytogenes, Salmonella* spp., *Shigella, Vibrio cholerae, Yersinia enterocolitica,* Aeromonas, *Bacillus cereus* (if HIV+ consider *Mycobacterium avium* complex)

Viruses: *Adenovirus, Astrovirus, Rotavirus, Norovirus (Norwalk)*

Protozoa: *Cryptosporidium, Cyclospora, Entamoeba histolytica, Giardia* (if HIV+ consider *Microsporidia*)

Empiric Therapy
(Treatment duration: 3–5 days)

- Azithromycin 500 mg (P 10 mg/kg) PO once daily
- Levofloxacin 500 mg PO once daily
- Ciprofloxacin 500 mg PO two times daily

Campylobacter Jejuni
(Treatment duration: 3–5 days, 7–14 days for immunocompromised patients)

- Treatment only recommended in severe cases

- Azithromycin 500 mg (Ⓟ 10 mg/kg) PO once daily for 3 days
- Levofloxacin 500 mg PO once daily
- Ciprofloxacin 500 mg PO two times daily

Clostridioides Difficile

- See Clostridioides Difficile Infections, p. 35

E. Coli O157:H7 and Shiga toxin-producing E. coli (STEC)

- Antibiotic treatment should be avoided as it may increase the risk of hemolytic uremic syndrome

Salmonella
(Treatment duration: 5–7 days, 14 days for immunocompromised)

- Routine treatment is not recommended
- May consider treatment for age < 3 months or > 50 yrs, or has prostheses, significant joint disease, valvular heart disease, severe atherosclerosis, malignancy, sickle cell, AAA, or uremia
  - Amoxicillin 500 mg (Ⓟ 10 mg/kg) PO three times daily
  - Levofloxacin 500 mg PO once daily
  - Ciprofloxacin 500 mg PO two times daily
  - Ceftriaxone 1 g (Ⓟ 50 mg/kg) IV once daily (consider 2 g if > 100 kg or severe infection)
- If concern for extensively resistant *Salmonella* Typhimurium (XDR)
  - Azithromycin 500 mg PO once daily

Shigella
(Treatment duration: 3 days unless otherwise noted; 7–10 days for immunocompromised patients)

- Azithromycin 500 mg (Ⓟ 10 mg/kg) PO daily
- Levofloxacin 500 mg PO once daily
- Ciprofloxacin 500 mg PO two times daily
- Ceftriaxone 1 g (Ⓟ 100 mg/kg) IV once daily for 5 days (consider 2 g if > 100 kg or severe infection)

Vibrio Cholerae
(Treatment duration: single dose)

- Doxycycline 300 mg PO once
- Azithromycin 1 g (Ⓟ 20 mg/kg) PO once
- Ciprofloxacin 1 g PO once

GI

Yersinia Enterocolitica
(Treatment duration: 5 days)

Note: Antibiotics are not indicated unless bacteremia is present

- TMP/SMX (DS) 1 tablet (ⓟ 4 mg/kg) PO two times daily
- Ciprofloxacin 500 mg PO two times daily
- Levofloxacin 500 mg PO once daily
- Ceftriaxone 1 g (ⓟ 100 mg/kg) IV once daily (consider 2 g if > 100 kg or severe infection)

Entamoeba Histolytica
- Metronidazole 750 mg PO three times daily for 5–10 days **PLUS:**
  - Paromomycin 500 mg PO three times daily for 7 days **OR**
  - Iodoquinol 650 mg PO three times daily for 20 days

Giardia Lamblia
- Tinidazole 2 g PO once
- Metronidazole 500 mg PO two times daily for 5–10 days
- Nitazoxanide 500 mg PO two times daily for 3 days

Cryptosporidium
- Nitazoxanide 500 mg PO two times daily for 3 days

PEARLS
- Indications for empiric therapy
  - Infant < 3 months old with suspected bacterial etiology
  - Ill-appearing with documented fever, abdominal pain, bloody diarrhea
  - Recent international travel with temperature > 38.4°C or signs of sepsis
- Consider local or regional resistance patterns when choosing an antibiotic because of increasing quinolone and sulfa resistance
- Avoid medications that decrease intestinal motility
- Consider stool testing if diarrhea is accompanied by fever, severe abdominal cramping, bloody or mucoid stools, or sepsis

PERITONEAL DIALYSIS-RELATED PERITONITIS

Common organisms: *Staphylococcus* spp., *Streptococcus* spp., *Enterococcus* spp., *Pseudomonas* spp., *Klebsiella* spp., *Enterobacter* spp., polymicrobial, anaerobes

Intraperitoneal (IP) Route (preferred)
■ Vancomycin 30 mg/kg IP **PLUS:**
  - Cefepime 1 g IP **OR**
  - Ceftriaxone 1 g IP (consider 2 g if > 100 kg or severe infection) **OR**
  - Gentamicin 0.6 mg/kg IP (*see weight-based dosing, p. 101*) **OR**
  - Aztreonam 2 g daily **OR**
  - Imipenem/cilastatin 500 mg IP in alternate exchange

IV Route
■ Vancomycin 15–20 mg/kg IV **PLUS:**
  - Cefepime 1 g IV **OR**
  - Imipenem/cilastatin 500 mg IV two times daily **OR**
  - Aztreonam 500 mg IV three times daily

PEARLS
■ Recommend consultation with ID and Nephrology
■ PD-related peritonitis diagnosed with any **TWO** of the following: abdominal pain and/or cloudy dialysis effluent, dialysis effluent > 100 WBC/mm^3 with > 50% PMNs, or positive effluent cultures
■ Consider treatment for fungal peritonitis if patient has received antibiotics for bacterial peritonitis in past 3 months or immunosuppression
■ Recommend initiating empiric treatment early if clinical suspicion high in the setting of cloudy dialysis effluent

GI

PERITONITIS/PERFORATED VISCUS/ INTRA-ABDOMINAL ABSCESS

Common organisms: Polymicrobial

Mild to Moderate Disease

- Metronidazole 500 mg (🅟 10 mg/kg) IV three times daily) **PLUS:**
    - Ceftriaxone 1 g (🅟 100 mg/kg) IV once daily (consider 2 g if > 100 kg) **OR**
    - Ciprofloxacin 400 mg IV two times daily **OR**
    - Levofloxacin 750 mg IV once daily
- Moxifloxacin 400 mg IV once daily
- Ertapenem 1 g IV once daily (🅟 15 mg/kg two times daily)

Severe/Life-Threatening Disease

- Metronidazole 500 mg (🅟 10 mg/kg) IV three times daily **AND** cefepime 2 g (🅟 50 mg/kg) IV three times daily
- Piperacillin/tazobactam 4.5 g (🅟 100 mg/kg) IV four times daily
- Imipenem/cilastatin 1 g IV three times daily (🅟 25 mg/kg IV four times daily)
- Meropenem 1 g (🅟 20 mg/kg) IV three times daily

SPONTANEOUS BACTERIAL PERITONITIS

Common organisms: *E. coli*, *Klebsiella* spp., *Streptococcus* spp., *Enterobacter* spp., *Enterococci* spp., *Staphylococcus* spp.

- Ceftriaxone 1 g IV once daily (consider 2 g if > 100 kg or severe infection)
- Piperacillin/tazobactam 4.5 g IV three times daily
- Ertapenem 1 g IV once daily

Prior Quinolone Prophylaxis

- **ADD** vancomycin 15–20 mg/kg IV two–three times daily to above

PEARLS

- SBP: > 250 PMN/mm^3 in the peritoneal fluid
- For patients with serum creatinine > 1 mg/dL, blood urea nitrogen > 30 mg/dL, or total bilirubin > 4 mg/dL, administer first dose of albumin 1.5 g/kg within 6 hrs of diagnosis to reduce hepatorenal syndrome and mortality

BACTERIAL VAGINOSIS

Common organisms: *Gardnerella* spp., polymicrobial
(Treatment duration: 7 days unless otherwise noted)

- Metronidazole 500 mg PO two times daily
- Metronidazole vaginal gel 0.75% one applicator (5 g) vaginally nightly for 5 days
- Clindamycin vaginal cream 2% one applicator (5 g) vaginally nightly
- Clindamycin 300 mg PO two times daily

PEARLS

- May substitute tinidazole 2 g PO daily for 2 days **OR** 1 g PO daily for 5 days in non-pregnant patients
- Single dose of metronidazole is no longer recommended
- Oral or vaginal regimens acceptable in pregnancy
- Insufficient evidence to support treatment in asymptomatic patients (including pregnancy and/or partner)

BALANITIS

Common organisms: *Candida* spp., occasionally *Staph* or *Streptococcus*, anaerobes

May be non-infectious (in men, 50% of cases): irritant, allergic, inflammatory, autoimmune, trauma, or malignancy

Initial Treatment (suspected *Candida* spp.)

- Careful cleansing of foreskin, sitz baths
- Clotrimazole 1% applied two times daily until symptoms resolve
- Miconazole 2% applied two times daily until symptoms resolve (7 days)
- Nystatin 100,000 units/g cream applied two times daily for imidazole resistance or allergy (14 days)
- Fluconazole 150 mg PO once (severe symptoms)

Suspected Anaerobes

(Erythema, edema, foul-smelling exudate)

- Metronidazole 500 mg PO two times daily for 7 days

Suspected Circinate Balanitis

(Pale macules with white margins that may coalesce; can occur in isolation or association with reactive arthritis)

- Hydrocortisone 1% twice daily for 7-14 days

GU

Suspected *Staphylococcus aureus* or *Streptococcus pyogenes*

(Intense erythema and transudative or exudative preputial discharge)

- Mupirocin 2% cream applied three times daily for 7-14 days
    - If more severe or phymosis prevents topical treatment:
        - Cephalexin 500 mg PO four times daily for 7 days **OR**
        - Clindamycin 450 mg PO three times daily for 7 days

PEARLS

- Distinguishing between infectious etiologies and STIs is critical, especially in prepubescent child who may be victim of sexual abuse: HIV, HSV, trichomonas, syphilis (screen for STD/STI when indicated)
- Non-infectious considerations: inflammatory skin disorders, lichen planus, psoriasis, lichen sclerosis, erythema multiforme, chemical irritants, diabetes, immunocompromised state, reactive arthritis, inadequate hygiene
- Balanitis that persists despite treatment mandates urologic follow-up (may represent cancerous/precancerous lesions)

ENDOMETRITIS

Common organisms: Often polymicrobial, including anaerobes, *C. trachomatis*, and *M. hominis*

Non-Obstetric

(Treatment duration: 14 days)

- Ceftriaxone 500 mg IM **AND** doxycycline 100 mg PO two times daily **AND** metronidazole 500 mg PO two times daily

Postpartum or Recent Gynecologic Procedure

- Gentamicin 5–7 mg/kg IV once daily (*see weight-based dosing, p. 101*) **PLUS:**
    - Clindamycin 900 mg IV three times daily **OR**
    - Ampicillin/sulbactam 3 g IV four times daily
- All three antibiotics recommended with known GBS colonization

PEARLS

- Obstetric endometritis more likely after c-section (especially anaerobic)
- Consider pelvic US for retained POC in postpartum endometritis
- Consider removal of intrauterine devices if no clinical improvement within 48–72 hrs of antibiotic initiation

EPIDIDYMITIS/ORCHITIS

Common organisms: STD/STI suspected: *N. gonorrhea*, *C. trachomatis*;
STD/STI NOT suspected: *Pseudomonas* spp., *E. coli*

Gonorrhea/chlamydia suspected
(Treatment duration: 10 days)
- Ceftriaxone 500 mg IM once **AND** doxycycline 100 mg PO two times daily for 10 days
- If severe PCN allergy:
  - Gentamicin 240 mg IM once **AND** azithromycin 2 g PO once

Recent GU procedure, BPH, or STD/STI not suspected
- Levofloxacin 500 mg PO once daily for 10 days (21 days if associated prostatitis)

Treat STD/STI and enteric organisms in men who practice anal sex
- Ceftriaxone 500 mg IM once **AND** levofloxacin 500 mg PO once daily for 10 days

PEARLS
- Etiology: bacterial, viral (eg, mumps), trauma, post-prostatic biopsy, post-vasectomy, exercise, prolonged sitting
- Consider CMV, *Salmonella*, mycobacteria, and fungi in HIV positive patients who do not respond to initial therapy
- Bacterial etiology is uncommon (< 6%) in children
- Consider testicular torsion and Fournier's gangrene
- Consider UA, UCx, and urine NAAT for *N. gonorrhea* and *C. trachomatis*
- If STD/STI suspected, sexual partners within 60 days should be treated
- Rest, ice, NSAIDs, and scrotal support are important adjuncts for pain
- Chronic epididymitis > 6 weeks, refer to urologist and consider TB risk factors

HERPES SIMPLEX VIRUS

First Episode
(Treatment duration: 7–10 days)
- Acyclovir 400 mg PO three times daily
- Valacyclovir 1 g PO two times daily
- Famciclovir 250 mg PO three times daily

GU

Recurrent Episode
- Acyclovir 800 mg PO three times daily for 2 days
- Valacyclovir 500 mg PO two times daily for 3 days
- Famciclovir 1 g PO two times daily for 1 day

HIV-Positive: First or recurrent episode
(Treatment duration: 5-10 days if orolabial disease; 7-10 days if genital disease unless recurrent episode, which is 5-10)
- Acyclovir 400 mg PO three times daily
- Valacyclovir 1 g PO two times daily
- Famciclovir 500 mg PO two times daily

Severe Disease or Complicated Course (disseminated infection, pneumonitis, hepatitis, meningitis, or encephalitis)
- Acyclovir 5-10 mg/kg IV three times daily (use ideal body weight unless encephalitis/meningitis — use adjusted body weight)
- Convert IV to PO therapy when lesions regress, then continue PO therapy until lesions have fully healed
- For acyclovir-resistant severe disease: foscarnet 40-80 mg/kg IV three times daily (use actual body weight)

Pregnant: Suppressive therapy recommended starting at 36 weeks gestation
- Acyclovir 400 mg PO three times daily
- Valacyclovir 500 mg PO two times daily

Neonates (Treatment duration: 14 days if disease is limited to skin and mucous membranes, 21 days for CNS involvement and disseminated disease)
- Acyclovir 20 mg/kg IV three times daily

PEARLS
- Caution: Antivirals as listed may require dose adjustment if renal insufficiency
- Alternative dosing regimens are available from the CDC

PELVIC INFLAMMATORY DISEASE

Common organisms: *N. gonorrhea, C. trachomatis, S. agalactiae, G. vaginalis*, enteric gram-negative rods, anaerobes

Outpatient
- Ceftriaxone 500 mg (1 g if > 150 kg) IM once **AND** doxycycline 100 mg PO two times daily for 14 days **AND** metronidazole 500 mg PO two times daily for 14 days

Inpatient

- Doxycycline 100 mg PO/IV two times daily **PLUS:**
  - Ceftriaxone 1 g IV once daily **AND** metronidazole 500 mg IV two times daily **OR**
  - Ampicillin-sulbactam 3 g IV four times daily
- Clindamycin 900 mg IV three times daily **AND** gentamicin 3–5 mg/kg IV once daily (*weight-based dosing*)
- In pregnancy, use ceftriaxone as dosed above **AND** azithromycin 1 g PO once in place of doxycycline

PEARLS

- Consider admission if:
  - Suspected TOA or pelvic abscess
  - Pregnancy
  - Nausea, vomiting, high fever, or failure of outpatient therapy
  - Any patient if compliance or follow-up is questionable
- Fluoroquinolones are no longer recommended because of rising levels of resistance among *N. gonorrhea* isolates (may be considered for outpatient regimen if true cephalosporin allergy)
- Consider testing the patient for syphilis, HIV
- Treat sexual partners within past 60 days (or most recent partner if contact was > 60 days prior)
- Abstain from intercourse until 7 days after therapy is initiated **AND** symptom resolution **AND** partners have been treated

PROSTATITIS

Common organisms: *E. coli, N. gonorrhea,* and *C. trachomatis*

STD/STI not suspected
(Treatment duration: 4–6 weeks; refer to local antibiogram)

- Ciprofloxacin 500 mg PO two times daily
- Levofloxacin 500 mg PO once daily
- TMP/SMX (DS) 1 tablet PO two times daily

STD/STI suspected
(Treatment duration: 14 days)

- Ceftriaxone 500 mg (1 g if > 150 kg) IM once **AND** doxycycline 100 mg PO two times daily

Severe infection (bacteremia, sepsis, or suspected prostatic abscess)

- Ceftriaxone 1 g IV once daily (consider 2 g if > 100 kg)
- Ciprofloxacin 400 mg IV two times daily
- Levofloxacin 500 mg IV once daily
- Ertapenem 1 g IV once daily

PEARLS

- Urine Gram stain and culture recommended in all men suspected of acute prostatitis
- Consider pseudomonal coverage (eg, cefepime) if recent instrumentation
- Total length of therapy should be 4–6 weeks if concern for chronic prostatitis
- If urinary retention due to prostatitis, consider urologic consultation before catheter placement

PYELONEPHRITIS

Common organisms: *E. coli, Enterococcus* spp., *Klebsiella* spp., *Proteus* spp., *S. saprophyticus*

Outpatient, Adults

- Cefpodoxime 200 mg PO two times daily for 10–14 days
- TMP/SMX (DS)* 1 tablet PO two times daily for 10–14 days
- Ciprofloxacin* 500 mg PO two times daily for 7 days
- Levofloxacin* 750 mg PO once daily for 5 days

*Note: Evaluate local susceptibilities; if local resistance > 10%, recommend initial dose of ceftriaxone or aminoglycoside. Utilize TMP/SMX, ciprofloxacin, or levofloxacin if culture data supports

Inpatient, Adult

Note: Begin with IV therapy and switch to PO once afebrile for 24–48 hrs

If not suspecting enterococcal infection

- Ceftriaxone 1 g IV once daily
- Ciprofloxacin 400 mg IV two times daily
- Levofloxacin 750 mg IV once daily
- Cefepime 2 g IV three times daily (*Pseudomonas* coverage)
- If severe PCN allergy:
  - Gentamicin 5 mg/kg IV once daily (*see weight-based dosing, p. 101*) **OR**
  - Aztreonam 2 g IV three times daily

If suspected or known enterococcal infection

- Ampicillin 2 g IV four times daily **PLUS/MINUS** gentamicin 1 mg/kg IV three times daily (*see weight-based dosing, p. 101*)

Pregnancy
(Treatment duration 10-14 days)

Outpatient
- ▣ Ceftriaxone 1 g IV once **PLUS:**
  - – If no recent ABx or history of resistance:
    - • Cephalexin 500 mg PO four times daily **OR**
    - • Cefadroxil 1 g PO two times daily
  - – If recent ABx exposure or concern for resistance:
    - • Cefpodoxime 200 mg PO two times daily

Inpatient
- ▣ Ceftriaxone 1 g IV daily **THEN** follow blood culture susceptibilities and choose antibiotic based on susceptibility and safety in pregnancy

Inpatient, Pediatric
Note: Begin with IV therapy, and switch to PO once afebrile for 48–72 hrs
- ▣ Ceftriaxone 100 mg/kg IV once daily
- ▣ Ampicillin 25 mg/kg IV four times daily **AND** gentamicin 2.5 mg/kg IV three times daily (*see weight-based dosing, p. 101*)

PEARLS
- ▣ In general, admit all pregnant patients with pyelonephritis
- ▣ Oral beta-lactam agents may be less effective than other options Recommend using an initial parenteral dose of a long-acting antimicrobial (eg, ceftriaxone or aminoglycoside)
- ▣ Patients with hypotension/shock, recurrent pyelonephritis, or persistent symptoms after 3 days of treatment should be imaged to rule out stone or perinephric abscess
- ▣ Pediatric patients should have urologic follow-up to rule out urinary tract malformations

SEXUAL ASSAULT STD/STI PROPHYLAXIS

Common organisms: *C. trachomatis, N. gonorrhea, Trichomonas* spp., Hepatitis B, HIV, HPV, tetanus

GC/Chlamydia/Trichomonas
- ▣ Ceftriaxone 500 mg (consider 1 g if > 150 kg) IM once **AND** doxycycline 100 mg PO two times daily for 7 days
  - – Consider replacing doxycycline with azithromycin 1 g PO once if compliance in question or pregnant

GU

- For female patients, **ADD** metronidazole 500 mg PO two times daily for 7 days (empiric treatment for trichomoniasis only indicated for female patients)
- Consider replacing metronidazole 500 mg PO two times daily with metronidazole 2 g PO once if compliance in question

HBV

- Hep B vaccination not indicated if known to be vaccinated and has documented immunity
- If vaccinated but uncertain immunity, give single dose of Hep B vaccine
- If unvaccinated: Should have post-exposure vaccination with initial dose given preferably within 24 hrs and **THEN** follow-up doses at 1–2 months and 6 months
- If unvaccinated or uncertain immunity and assailant is known to be HBV infected: HBIG is also recommended (see *Occupational Post-Exposure, p. 82*)

HIV

- HIV non-occupational PEP (nPEP) should be considered in certain situations if assault occurred within 72 hrs of evaluation
- National Clinician's PEP Hotline: 888-448-4911

HPV

- If not already vaccinated, may initiate the series and/or refer to PCP for vaccination series
- All patients aged 9–26 years
- Consider in selected patients age 27–45 years (new or multiple sexual partners)

Tetanus exposure: See *Tetanus, p. 78*

PEARLS

- Serologic testing for syphilis and HIV also recommended by the CDC
- Consider pregnancy prophylaxis: levonorgestrel 1.5 mg PO once **OR** ulipristal 30 mg PO once up to 5 days post assault **OR** copper IUD up to 5 days post-assault or post-ovulation, whichever is longer
- Consider tetanus prophylaxis

SYPHILIS

Common organism: *T. pallidum*

Primary/Secondary/Early Latent Syphilis

Early latent = acquired in past year

- Benzathine penicillin G 2.4 million units (P 50,000U/kg) IM once
- If severe PCN allergy:
  - Doxycycline 100 mg PO two times daily for 14 days

Tertiary Syphilis/Late Latent Syphilis/Syphilis of Unknown Duration
Late latent = likely acquired > 1 year prior
- Benzathine penicillin G 2.4 million units (ⓟ 50,000U/kg) IM once a week for 3 weeks
- If severe PCN allergy: doxycycline 100 mg PO two times daily for 28 days

Neurosyphilis/Ocular Syphilis
- Aqueous crystalline penicillin G 3–4 million units IV six times daily for 10–14 days
- Procaine penicillin G 2.4 million units IM daily **AND** probenecid 500 mg PO four times daily for 10–14 days

PEARLS
- Penicillin G is treatment of choice; limited data on efficacy of other regimens
- Treated patients should abstain from sexual activity for 7 days following treatment completion
- Pregnant and neurosyphilis patients allergic to penicillin should be desensitized and treated with penicillin
- Sexual partners from 90 days preceding diagnosis should receive empiric primary syphilis treatment
- All sexual partners should have serologic testing performed
- Counsel patients on potential Jarisch-Herxheimer reaction (rigors, fever, myalgia), typically within first 24 hrs of treatment
- Recommend LP for ocular complaints, neurologic symptoms, or HIV positive
- All patients presenting with syphilis should be tested for HIV
- Children > 1 month—if not congenital, consider evaluation for sexual abuse

TRICHOMONIASIS

Initial or Reinfection
- Metronidazole 500 mg PO two times daily for 7 days (women); metronidazole 2 g PO once (men)
- Tinidazole 2 g PO once

Persistent
- Metronidazole 2 g PO daily for 7 days **OR** tinidazole 2 g PO daily for 7 days (women); metronidazole 500 mg PO two daily 7 days (men)

PEARLS
- No true effective alternatives to nitroimidazole therapy; therefore IgE mediated allergic patients should be desensitized

GU

- Sexual partners should be treated; sexually active women should be retested 3 months after completing treatment because of high reinfection rates
- Avoid breastfeeding for 24 hrs after the last dose of metronidazole or 72 hrs after the last dose of tinidazole
- Alcohol avoidance no longer necessary
- Preferred regimen in children is metronidazole 15 mg/kg PO three times daily for 7 days; evaluate for sexual abuse

URETHRITIS/CERVICITIS

Co-infection is common with gonorrhea and chlamydia; treat for both

Common organisms: *N. gonorrhea, C. trachomatis, U. urealyticum, M. genitalium, Trichomonas* spp., HSV

- Ceftriaxone 500 mg (1 g if > 150 kg) IM once **AND** doxycycline 100 mg PO two times daily for 7 days
  - Consider replacing doxycycline with azithromycin 1 g PO once if compliance in question or pregnant

If severe PCN or cephalosporin allergy:

- Azithromycin 2 g PO once **AND** gentamicin 240 mg IM once
  - Anti-emetic recommended with high-dose azithromycin

PEARLS

- Treat known sexual partners within past 60 days (or most recent partner if contact was > 60 days prior)
- Abstain from intercourse until 7 days after therapy is initiated **AND** symptom resolution **AND** partners have been treated
- Fluoroquinolones are no longer recommended for treatment of gonococcal urethritis because of rising levels of resistance among *N. gonorrhoeae* isolates
- Although thought to be less effective, cefixime 800 mg PO once may be considered as a replacement when IM ceftriaxone is not an option
- Retesting at 3 months recommended because of high recurrence rates
- Consider testing patient for other STD/STI such as HIV and syphilis
- Consider treatment with metronidazole for *Trichomonas* spp. and/or bacterial vaginosis infection, especially in resistant cases
- Test of cure recommended 3–4 weeks later for pregnant women and at 14 days for individuals receiving an alternative regimen

URINARY TRACT INFECTION (UTI)/CYSTITIS

CHOOSING WISELY RECOMMENDATIONS
- ▨ Do NOT obtain a urine culture unless there are clear signs and symptoms that localize to the urinary tract
- ▨ Do NOT treat asymptomatic bacteriuria with antibiotics (except in pregnancy)
- ▨ Avoid using a fluoroquinolone for first-line treatment of uncomplicated UTIs

ADULT

Uncomplicated UTI (dysuria, frequency, or urgency in otherwise healthy, non-pregnant female patients)

Common organisms: *E. coli, Klebsiella* spp., *P. mirabilis, S. saprophyticus*

- ▨ Beta-lactam (Treatment duration: 5–7 days)
  - Cephalexin 500 mg PO two times daily
  - Cefuroxime 500 mg PO two times daily
  - Cefpodoxime 100 mg PO two times daily (*more expensive*)
- ▨ Nitrofurantoin 100 mg PO two times daily for 5 days (avoid if pyelonephritis suspected or CrCl < 30 mL/min)
- ▨ TMP/SMX (DS) 1 tablet PO two times daily for 3–5 days (consider alternative if local *E. coli* resistance > 20%)
- ▨ Fosfomycin 3 g PO once
- ▨ Fluoroquinolone (Treatment duration: 3 days) **Consider FDA warning on risk vs. benefit**
  - Ciprofloxacin 250 mg PO two times daily
  - Levofloxacin 250 mg PO once daily

Complicated UTI (male patients, patients with obstruction, immunosuppression, renal transplantation, indwelling catheter/stent, urologic dysfunction, urinary retention)

Common organisms: *E. coli, Klebsiella* spp., *Proteus* spp., *Pseudomonas* spp., *Enterococcus* spp.

- ▨ Beta-lactam (Treatment duration: 7–10 days)
  - No recent ABx exposure and low risk for resistance: cephalexin 500 mg PO four times daily
  - Cefuroxime 500 mg PO two times daily
  - Cefpodoxime 200 mg PO two times daily
  - Cefazolin 1 g IV three times daily
  - Ceftriaxone 1 g IV daily
  - Cefepime 2 g IV three times daily (reserve for *Pseudomonas* spp.)
  - Imipenem/cilastatin 1 g IV three times daily (reserve for multi-drug

resistant pathogens)
- TMP/SMX (DS) 1 tablet PO two times daily for 7–10 days (consider alternative if local *E. coli* resistance > 20%)
- Fosfomycin 3 g PO every 48 hrs for 3 doses (reserve for multi-drug resistant pathogens)
- Gentamicin 5 mg/kg IV once daily (*see weight-based dosing, p. 101*)
- Fluoroquinolone **(Consider FDA warning on risk vs. benefit)**
  - Ciprofloxacin 500 mg PO two times daily **OR** 400 mg IV two times daily for 7 days
  - Levofloxacin 750 mg PO/IV once daily for 5 days

Pregnant
- Asymptomatic bacteriuria: cephalexin 500 mg PO three times daily for 4-7 days
- No recent ABx exposure or history of ABx resistance:
  - Cephalexin 500 mg PO four times daily for 7 days
  - Cefadroxil 1 g PO two times daily for 7 days
- Recent ABx exposure or concern for resistance:
  - Cefpodoxime 200 mg PO two times daily for 7 days
- Fosfomycin 3 g PO once every 48 hrs for 3 doses
- Nitrofurantoin 100 mg PO two times daily **OR** TMP/SMX (DS) 1 tablet PO two times daily
  - **AVOID during first trimester** unless there is no therapeutic alternative
  - **AVOID** in patients > 36 weeks gestation because of increased risk of neonatal hemolytic anemia (nitrofurantoin) or kernicterus (sulfonamides)

PEARLS
- Consider recent urine culture data to guide empiric antibiotic choice

PEDIATRIC

Pediatric Outpatient
(Treatment duration: 5 days if > 2 years and first UTI;
7–14 days if history of UTIs or age < 2 years)
- Cephalexin 25 mg/kg PO four times daily
- Cefdinir 14 mg/kg PO once daily
- Amoxicillin/clavulanate 10 mg/kg PO three times daily (dose based on amoxicillin component)
- TMP/SMX 4 mg/kg PO two times daily (dose based on TMP component)

Pediatric Inpatient
- Ceftriaxone 75 mg/kg IV once daily
- Gentamicin 2.5 mg/kg IV three times daily (*see weight-based dosing, p. 101*)

GU

VULVOVAGINAL CANDIDIASIS

Intravaginal Therapy for Uncomplicated Candidal Vaginitis (preparations available OTC)

- Clotrimazole 1% cream one applicator vaginally for 7–14 nights **OR** 2% cream one applicator vaginally for 3 nights
- Miconazole 2% cream one applicator vaginally for 7 nights **OR** 4% cream one applicator vaginally for 3 nights
- Miconazole 100 mg one suppository vaginally for 7 nights **OR** 200 mg one suppository vaginally for 3 nights
- Miconazole 1200 mg one suppository vaginally once
- Tioconazole 6.5% ointment one applicator vaginally once

Intravaginal Therapy for Uncomplicated Candidal Vaginitis (prescription)

- Terconazole 80 mg one suppository vaginally for 3 nights **OR** 0.8% cream vaginally for 3 nights **OR** 0.4% cream vaginally for 7 days
- Butoconazole 2% cream one applicator vaginally once (do not use during first trimester of pregnancy)

Oral Therapy for Vulvovaginal Candidiasis

- Fluconazole 150 mg PO once (may repeat in 72 hrs if symptoms persist)
  — **Note:** concern for increased risk of miscarriage in pregnancy

PEARLS

- Only topical imidazole (clotrimazole, miconazole) therapy, applied for 7 days, is recommended in pregnancy
- Severe VVC (extensive vulvar erythema, edema, excoriation, or fissure formation) or immunocompromised host should be treated with 7–14 days of topical azole or two sequential oral doses of 150 mg fluconazole 72 hrs apart
- No treatment of sexual partner needed. A minority of male sex partners may have balanitis in conjunction with pruritus and irritation and may benefit from topical treatment
- Creams and suppositories are oil-based and may weaken latex condoms or diaphragms; advise patient to refer to condom product labelling for details

GU

ACUTE EXACERBATION OF CHRONIC BRONCHITIS (AECB)/COPD

Common organisms: Viral (Rhinovirus, RSV, influenza/parainfluenza), *H. influenzae, S. pneumoniae, M. catarrhalis, Pseudomonas* spp., *Enterobacteriaceae, C. pneumoniae, M. pneumoniae*

Outpatient

(Treatment duration: 5–7 days unless otherwise noted)

- Amoxicillin-clavulanate 875 mg PO two times daily for 5 days
- Azithromycin 500 mg PO once daily for 3 days
- Azithromycin 500 mg PO once, **THEN** 250 mg PO once daily for 4 days
- Cefuroxime 500 mg PO two times daily
- TMP/SMX (DS) 1 tablet PO two times daily

Inpatient

- Ceftriaxone 1 g IV once daily (consider 2 g if > 100 kg or severe infection)
- Moxifloxacin 400 mg PO/IV once daily
- If *Pseudomonas* spp. suspected:*
  - Cefepime 2 g IV three times per day
  - Piperacillin/tazobactam 4.5 g IV four times daily
  - Levofloxacin 750 mg PO/IV once daily

PEARLS

- Cardinal symptoms of AECB: increased dyspnea, increased sputum volume, increased sputum purulence
- Antibiotics should be given if 3 cardinal symptoms are present or increased sputum is present with one additional cardinal symptom
- Patients on mechanical ventilation for AECB should receive antibiotics
- Choice of antibiotics should be guided by local bacterial resistance pattern
- Adjunctive treatment: short-acting anticholinergic bronchodilators and inhaled beta-2 agonists along with corticosteroids
- *Pseudomonas* spp. risk factors: bronchiectasis, multiple recent antibiotics, frequent hospitalizations, chronic oral steroid use

PULMONARY

BRONCHITIS

PEARLS

- Vast majority (> 90%) of cases are caused by viruses
- Symptomatic treatment: rest, antitussive (benzonatate, guaifenesin), and bronchodilators may be helpful in adults
- Antibiotics are **not** the mainstay of treatment and may increase adverse events and antimicrobial resistance
- Antibiotics are recommended for acute exacerbation of chronic bronchitis
- During influenza season, consider influenza infection and antiviral medications for high-risk patients who present within 48 hrs
- Consider pertussis in patients with prolonged cough and inquire about close contacts with viral symptoms; if suspected, a macrolide antibiotic is recommended
- Mycoplasma pneumonia may cause prolonged cough in children > 5 yrs old

INFLUENZA

Note: **Antiviral treatment recommended for patients requiring hospitalization, those with severe, complicated, or progressive illness, or immunocompromised**

Influenza A & B
- Oseltamivir
  (Treatment duration: 5 days)
  - Adult: 75 mg PO two times daily
    - CrCl 30–60 mL/min: 30 mg PO two times daily
    - CrCl 10–30 mL/min: 30 mg PO once daily
  - Ⓟ Pediatric
    - 2 weeks–1 year: 3 mg/kg/dose PO two times daily
    - Age > 1 year:
      - ≤ 15 kg: 30 mg PO two times daily
      - 15–23 kg: 45 mg PO two times daily
      - 24–40 kg: 60 mg PO two times daily
      - > 40 kg: 75 mg PO two times daily

PEARLS

- Outpatient treatment may decrease duration of illness by 1 day if started within 48 hrs of symptom onset (weigh against side effects such as nausea, vomiting, and rare neuropsychiatric events)
- Pregnant (up to 2 weeks postpartum): CDC recommends treatment

PULMONARY

- For control of outbreaks in institutional setting, CDC recommends prophylaxis for a minimum of 2 weeks and continuing up to 1 week after the last known case was identified regardless of vaccination status
- COVID-19 guidance: Consult the latest IDSA recommendations

COMMUNITY ACQUIRED PNEUMONIA (ADULT-OUTPATIENT)

Common organisms: *S. pneumoniae, H. influenzae, M. pneumoniae, C. pneumoniae*, viruses

No comorbidities or low risk for *P. aeruginosa* or MRSA
(no prior respiratory isolation, recent hospitalization, **NOR** IV antibiotics in previous 90 days)

- Amoxicillin 1 g PO three times daily for 5 days
- Doxycycline 100 mg PO two times daily for 5 days
- Azithromycin 500 mg PO once, **THEN** 250 mg PO once daily for 4 days (if local pneumococcal resistance is < 25%)

Significant comorbidities (chronic heart, lung, liver, or renal disease, diabetes, EtOH, active cancer, immunosuppression, asplenia)
Combination therapy

- Amoxicillin/clavulanate 875 mg PO two times daily (2 g PO two times daily of extended release formulation) **OR** cefpodoxime 200 mg PO two times daily **OR** cefuroxime 500 mg PO two times daily **PLUS:**
    - Azithromycin 500 mg PO once, **THEN** 250 mg PO once daily for 4 days **OR**
    - Doxycycline 100 mg PO two times daily for 5 days
- If severe PCN allergy:
    - Levofloxacin 750 mg PO daily for 5 days **OR**
    - Moxifloxacin 400 mg PO daily for 5 days

COMMUNITY ACQUIRED PNEUMONIA (ADULT-INPATIENT)

Common organisms: *S. pneumoniae, H. influenzae, M. pneumoniae, C. pneumoniae, Legionella* spp., viruses. *S. aureus* (including MRSA) may be considered in patients with necrotizing/cavitary infiltrate or empyema or patients with concurrent bacterial pneumonia in the setting of influenza

Inpatient, Non-severe

- Ceftriaxone 1 g IV once daily (consider 2 g if > 100 kg or severe infection) **PLUS:**
  - Doxycycline 100 mg PO/IV two times daily **OR**
  - Azithromycin 500 mg PO/IV once daily
- Levofloxacin 750 mg PO/IV once daily
- If history of respiratory MRSA infection in past year:
  - **ADD** vancomycin 25–30 mg/kg IV loading dose, **THEN** 15–20 mg/kg IV two–three times daily
- If history of *Pseudomonas aeruginosa* respiratory infection in past year, **REPLACE** ceftriaxone above with cefepime 2 g IV three times daily **OR** monotherapy with levofloxacin 750 mg IV once daily; review past culture data or local antibiogram and adjust accordingly

Severe pneumonia defined as either ONE major criterion OR ≥ 3 minor criteria	
Major criteria	**Minor criteria**
Septic shock with need for vasopressors	Respiratory rate ≥ 30 BPM
	PaO2/FIO2 ≤ 250
Respiratory failure requiring mechanical ventilation	Multilobar infiltrates
	Confusion/disorientation
	Uremia (BUN ≥ 20 mg/dL)
	Leukopenia due to infection (WBC < 4,000 cells/μL)
	Hypothermia (core temperature < 36°C)
	Hypotension requiring aggressive fluid resuscitation

Inpatient, Severe WITHOUT recent hospitalization AND no IV antibiotics in previous 90 days

- Ceftriaxone 1 g IV once daily (consider 2 g if > 100 kg or severe infection) **AND** azithromycin 500 mg IV once daily
- If severe PCN allergy:
  - Levofloxacin 750 mg IV once daily **OR**
  - Moxifloxacin 400 mg IV once daily
- If history of respiratory MRSA infection in past year:
  - **ADD** vancomycin 25–30 mg/kg IV loading dose, **THEN** 15–20 mg/kg IV two–three times daily
- If history of *Pseudomonas aeruginosa* respiratory infection in past year, **REPLACE** ceftriaxone above with cefepime 2 g IV three times daily **OR** monotherapy with levofloxacin 750 mg IV daily; review past culture data or local antibiogram and adjust accordingly

PULMONARY

Inpatient, Severe PLUS recent hospitalization AND IV ABx in prior 90 days

- Azithromycin 500 mg IV once daily **AND** vancomycin 25–30 mg/kg IV loading dose, **THEN** 15–20 mg/kg IV two–three times daily **PLUS:**
  - Cefepime 2 g IV three times daily **OR**
  - Piperacillin/tazobactam 4.5 g IV four times daily **OR**
  - Meropenem 1 g IV three times daily
- If severe PCN allergy:
  - Vancomycin 25–30 mg/kg IV loading dose, **THEN** 15–20 mg/kg IV two times daily **PLUS:**
    - Levofloxacin 750 mg IV once daily **OR**
    - Azithromycin 500 mg IV once daily **AND** aztreonam 2 g IV three times daily

PEARLS

- If clinically suspected, consider treatment for influenza if pregnant, hospitalized, or within 48 hrs of symptom onset
- For HIV positive or immunosuppressed patients
  - If CD4 count normal or > 200 cells/mm^3 treat as CA-pneumonia
  - CD4 count < 200 or clinical AIDS, see *Pneumocystis jiroveci* pneumonia, p. 80

ASPIRATION WITH LUNG ABSCESS/EMPYEMA

Note: Most patients with suspected aspiration do not require antibiotics; expect clinical resolution within 24-48 hrs. Prophylactic antibiotics have not been shown to improve outcomes in aspiration

Common organisms: Oral flora including *Streptococcus* spp., anaerobes, gram-negative spp.
- Ampicillin/sulbactam 3 g IV four times daily
- Ceftriaxone 1 g IV once daily (consider 2 g if > 100 kg or severe infection) **PLUS:**
  - Metronidazole 500 mg IV two times daily **OR**
  - Clindamycin 600 mg IV three times daily
- If severe PCN allergy:
  - Levofloxacin 750 mg IV once daily **PLUS:**
    - Metronidazole 500 mg IV two times daily **OR**
    - Clindamycin 600 mg IV three times daily
  - Moxifloxacin 400 mg IV once daily

PEARLS

- HCAP is no longer recognized and the diagnosis has been abandoned
- VAP: pneumonia that occurs 48 hrs after endotracheal intubation; treatment should be based on local or hospital guidelines
- If prior ESBL-producing gram-negative bacillus history, consider imipenem or meropenem
- Vancomycin plus piperacillin/tazobactam has increased risk of acute kidney injury

PULMONARY

PNEUMONIA (PEDIATRIC)

Outpatient

Common organisms: Respiratory syncytial virus, Influenza, *S. pneumoniae*, *H. influenzae*, *M. pneumoniae*, *C. pneumoniae*, other viruses

Presumed Bacterial Pneumonia
(Treatment duration: 7 days)
- Amoxicillin 45 mg/kg PO two times daily
- Amoxicillin/clavulanate 45 mg/kg PO two times daily (if NOT fully immunized)
- Cefpodoxime 5 mg/kg PO two times daily
- If severe PCN allergy:
  - Azithromycin 10 mg/kg PO once, **THEN** 5 mg/kg PO once daily **OR**
  - Levofloxacin 10 mg/kg PO
    - 6 months to 5 years: two times daily (max 750 mg/day)
    - > 5 years: once daily (max 750 mg/day)

Presumed Atypical Pneumonia
- Azithromycin 10 mg/kg PO once, **THEN** 5 mg/kg PO once daily for 4 days
- Doxycycline 1–2 mg/kg PO two times daily (> 7 years old) for 10–14 days

Inpatient

Common organisms: *S. pneumoniae, M. pneumoniae, C. pneumoniae, H. influenzae, M. catarrhalis, Legionella* spp., *E. coli, K. pneumoniae,* drug-resistant *S. aureus, Pseudomonas* spp., influenza, other viruses

Presumed Bacterial Pneumonia

Fully immunized with conjugate vaccines for *H. influenzae* type b and *S. pneumoniae*; local penicillin resistance in invasive strains of pneumococcus is minimal
- Ampicillin 50 mg/kg IV four times daily
- Ceftriaxone 50 mg/kg IV two times daily (max dose 2 g/day)
  - If < 44 weeks corrected gestational age, use cefotaxime 50 mg/kg three times daily in place of ceftriaxone
- If MRSA suspected **ADD** vancomycin 15 mg/kg IV four times daily

Not fully immunized for *H. influenzae* type b and *S. pneumoniae*; local penicillin resistance in invasive strains of pneumococcus is significant
- Ceftriaxone 50 mg/kg IV two times daily
- If severe PCN allergy: levofloxacin 10 mg/kg PO/IV
  - 6 months to 5 years: two times daily (max 750 mg/day)
  - > 5 years: once daily (max 750 mg/day)
- If MRSA suspected **ADD** vancomycin 15 mg/kg IV four times daily

PULMONARY

Abscess or Necrotizing Pneumonia

- **ADD** metronidazole 10 mg/kg/dose IV three times daily to above regimens

Presumed Atypical Pneumonia

- Preferred: azithromycin 10 mg/kg IV once daily for 2 days, **THEN** 5 mg/kg IV once daily for 4 days
- Doxycycline 1–2 mg/kg PO/IV two times daily (> 7 years old)
- Levofloxacin 10 mg/kg PO
  - 6 months to 5 years: two times daily (max 750 mg/day)
  - > 5 years: once daily (max 750 mg)

PEARLS

- Consider testing for influenza or other viral pathogens in the appropriate clinical setting as it may reduce unnecessary antimicrobial use
- Consider hospitalization in children < 6 months old with suspected bacterial community acquired pneumonia
- Consider supportive care only for children < 5 yrs, as etiology commonly viral

TUBERCULOSIS

Note: This is a reportable disease. Contact state and local health departments, and consult ID for dosing.

Common organisms: *Mycobacterium tuberculosis*

- **Drug-resistant TB:** studies are underway to test new treatments; current regimen depends on local sensitivities
- **Drug-susceptible TB:** a four-drug regimen over a 4-month period currently recommended: rifapentine, isoniazid, pyrazinamide, and moxifloxacin

PEARLS

- Patients under evaluation for TB should be placed in negative pressure isolation with airborne precautions
- High-risk patients for active infection
  - Immunocompromised
  - Recent prolonged exposure in endemic areas
  - Health care workers
  - History of IV drug use
- Concerning symptoms: cough > 3 weeks duration +/- hemoptysis, dyspnea; anorexia, fatigue, pleuritic chest pain; fever, night sweats
- Latent TB Infection (LTBI) screening
  - Two primary testing options: tuberculin skin test (TST) and Interferon-gamma release assays (IGRAs - preferred) for LTBI

ANIMAL/HUMAN BITE WOUNDS

Animal Bites

Key organisms: *Pasteurella* spp. (cat), *Streptococcus* spp., *Staphylococcus* spp., *Capnocytophaga canimorsus* (dog)
(Treatment duration: 7–10 days)

Oral Therapy

- ▪ Amoxicillin/clavulanate 875 mg/125 mg (Ⓟ 25 mg/kg) PO two times daily
- ▪ Cefuroxime 500 mg (Ⓟ 15 mg/kg) PO two times daily **AND** metronidazole 500 mg (Ⓟ 10 mg/kg) PO three times daily
- ▪ Moxifloxacin 400 mg PO once daily
- ▪ Clindamycin 300 mg (Ⓟ 10 mg/kg) PO three times daily **PLUS:**
  - – TMP/SMX (DS) 1–2 tablets (Ⓟ 5 mg/kg) PO two times daily **OR**
  - – Ciprofloxacin 500 mg (Ⓟ 15 mg/kg) PO two times daily **OR**
  - – Doxycycline 100 mg (Ⓟ 2 mg/kg) PO two times daily (> 7 yrs old)
    - • Acceptable in short courses (< 14 days) for all ages when necessary
- ▪ If severe PCN allergy **AND** pregnant:
  - – Azithromycin 500 mg PO once **THEN** 250 mg PO once daily for 4 days (high failure rate, variable activity against *Pasteurella* spp. and *Fusobacteria*)

IV Therapy

- ▪ Ampicillin/sulbactam 3 g (Ⓟ 50 mg/kg) IV four times daily
- ▪ Ceftriaxone 1 g (Ⓟ 50 mg/kg) IV once daily (consider 2 g if > 100 kg or severe infection) **AND** metronidazole 500 mg (Ⓟ 10 mg/kg) IV three times daily
- ▪ Clindamycin 600 mg (Ⓟ 10 mg/kg) IV three times daily **PLUS:**
  - – Ciprofloxacin 400 mg (Ⓟ 10 mg/kg) IV two times daily **OR**
  - – TMP/SMX 5 mg/kg IV two times daily

Human Bites

Key organisms: *Viridans* group streptococci, *Bacteroides* spp., coagulase-negative staphylococci, *Corynebacterium* spp., *S. aureus*, *Eikenella corrodens*, *Fusobacterium* spp., *Peptostreptococcus* spp.
(Treatment duration: 7–10 days)

- ▪ Amoxicillin/clavulanate 875 mg (Ⓟ 25 mg/kg) PO two times daily
- ▪ Moxifloxacin 400 mg PO once daily
- ▪ Clindamycin 450 mg (Ⓟ 10 mg/kg) PO three times daily **OR** metronidazole 500 mg (Ⓟ 10 mg/kg) PO three times daily **PLUS:**
  - – Doxycycline 100 mg (Ⓟ 2 mg/kg) PO two times daily (> 7 years old) **OR**
  - – Cefuroxime 500 mg (Ⓟ 15 mg/kg) PO two times daily **OR**
  - – Ciprofloxacin 500 mg (Ⓟ 15 mg/kg) PO two times daily **OR**
  - – TMP/SMX (DS) 1–2 tablets (Ⓟ 5 mg/kg) PO two times daily

SKIN & SOFT TISSUE

IV Therapy

- Ampicillin/sulbactam 3 g ((P) 50 mg/kg) IV four times daily
- Ceftriaxone 1 g ((P) 50 mg/kg) IV once daily (consider 2 g if > 100 kg or severe infection) **AND** metronidazole 500 mg ((P) 10 mg/kg) IV three times daily
- Moxifloxacin 400 mg IV once daily
- Clindamycin 600 mg ((P) 10 mg/kg) IV three times daily **AND** ciprofloxacin 400 mg ((P) 10 mg/kg) IV two times daily

PEARLS

- 3–5 days of prophylaxis is recommended for the following: edema or crush injury, immunocompromised or asplenic patients, advanced liver disease, all puncture wounds, all cat bite wounds, injuries that penetrate the periosteum or joint capsule, all facial, hand, foot, and genital area wounds
- Obtain radiographs if indicated
- Never close puncture wounds. Consider primary closure for facial wounds and loose approximation elsewhere
- Rabies and tetanus prophylaxis if indicated
- Consider Hepatitis B and HIV prophylaxis in human bites if high risk
- Indications for parenteral (IV) antibiotics include: systemic signs of toxicity, deep infection, rapid progression of erythema, progression of clinical findings after 48 hrs of oral ABx therapy, inability to tolerate oral therapy, proximity to indwelling device; consider in immunocompromised
- Short courses (< 14 days) of doxycycline acceptable for all ages when necessary

BARTHOLIN'S CYST/ABSCESS

Common organisms: Polymicrobial, *E. coli*, *S. aureus* (including MRSA), vaginal flora, *N. gonorrhoeae*, *C. trachomatis*, *B. fragilis*

- Incision and drainage with Word catheter placement or gauze packing is the mainstay of treatment
- Antimicrobial therapy typically **NOT** indicated
- Indications for ABx: surrounding cellulitis, recurrent infection, systemic signs of infection, immunosuppression, pregnancy, or concurrent STI

PEARLS

- Word catheter should be left in place as long as possible to promote tract formation
- Sitz baths assist with drainage
- OB-GYN follow-up for recurrent cases (for marsupialization) or perimenopausal patients (possible biopsy)
- In high-risk groups, consider culture of abscess and further evaluation for and treatment of STD/STI

SKIN & SOFT TISSUE

CELLULITIS AND ABSCESS

Nonpurulent (Cellulitis/Erysipelas)

Common organisms: Predominantly *Streptococcus* spp.
(Treatment duration: 5–7 days)

Outpatient

- Cephalexin 500 mg (ⓟ 6.25 mg/kg) PO four times daily
- Cefuroxime 500 mg (ⓟ 15 mg/kg) PO two times daily
- Cefadroxil 1 g PO once daily (ⓟ 15 mg/kg PO two times daily)
- If severe PCN allergy:
  - Clindamycin 450 mg (ⓟ 10 mg/kg) PO three times daily

Inpatient

- Cefazolin 1–2 g (ⓟ 30 mg/kg) IV three times daily
- If MRSA suspected or cannot tolerate cefazolin: vancomycin 15–20 mg/kg IV two–three times daily (ⓟ 10 mg/kg IV four times daily)

Purulent (Simple Cutaneous Abscess, Carbuncle, Furuncle, Cellulitis)

Common organisms: predominantly *Staphylococcus* spp. (including MSSA and CA-MRSA)

CHOOSING WISELY: I&D is treatment of choice; data on antibiotic use is controversial

Outpatient

Mild (adequate drainage and no systemic symptoms)

- No antibiotics

Moderate (Treatment duration: 5 days)

- TMP/SMX (DS) 1–2 tablets (ⓟ 5 mg/kg) PO two times daily
- Clindamycin 450 mg (ⓟ 10 mg/kg) PO three times daily
- Doxycycline 100 mg PO two times daily

Inpatient (Treatment duration: 5 days)

- Vancomycin 15–20 mg/kg IV two–three times daily (ⓟ 10 mg/kg IV four times daily)

PEARLS

- There is no evidence to support the practice of giving one dose of IV antibiotics prior to a course of outpatient oral antibiotics
- Consider imaging if concern for complicated soft tissue infection, including presence of gas or foreign bodies
- Consideration for newer glycopeptides (dalbavancin or oritavancin) may be appropriate in certain clinical situations (non-compliance, lack of follow-up, etc.) to avoid hospitalization

Water Exposure

Common organisms: *Aeromonas* spp.
(Treatment duration: 10 days with close follow-up)
- Cephalexin 500 mg PO four times daily
- If severe PCN allergy:
  - Clindamycin 450 mg PO or 600 mg IV (P 10 mg/kg) three times daily **AND** levofloxacin 750 mg IV/PO daily
- For sewage-contaminated water:
  - **ADD** metronidazole 500 mg PO three times daily

Saltwater Exposure

Common organisms: *Vibrio vulnificus*
(Treatment duration: 10 days)
- Ciprofloxacin 750 mg PO or 400 mg IV two times daily
- Doxycycline 100 mg PO/IV two times daily **AND** ceftriaxone 1 g IV daily (consider 2 g if > 100 kg or severe infection) for necrotizing infections
- Consider surgical consultation for severe soft tissue infection

Hidradenitis Suppurativa

(Refer to surgeon for definitive treatment)
- Single abscess without tract
  - Clindamycin 1% topical lotion applied to affected area two times daily until resolved
- Single/Multiple/Recurrent with tract
  - Doxycycline 100 mg PO two times daily
  - Clindamycin 300–450 mg PO three times daily

PEARLS
- Often patients with hidradenitis require several months of therapy
- Consider adding rifampin to oral clindamycin in consultation with ID

Perirectal Abscess

Common organisms: *Enterobacteriaceae*, *Bacteroides* spp., *Enterococcus* spp. (polymicrobial including gram-negative and anaerobic coverage)
Note: I&D is the treatment of choice. Recommend 5–10 days of empiric antibiotic coverage following I&D

Empiric/Uncomplicated
- Metronidazole 500 mg PO two times daily **PLUS:**
  - Cefpodoxime 400 mg PO two times daily **OR**
  - Ciprofloxacin 500 mg PO two times daily

= Pediatric dosing

Complicated (surrounding cellulitis, systemic symptoms, failure to improve with drainage alone)

- ▨ Metronidazole 500 mg PO/IV three times daily **PLUS:**
  - – Ceftriaxone 1 g IV once daily (consider 2 g if > 100 kg or severe infection) **OR**
  - – Levofloxacin 750 mg PO/IV once daily
- ▨ If MRSA suspected:
  - – **ADD** vancomycin 15–20 mg/kg IV two–three times daily

DIABETIC ULCERS

Common organisms: *Staphylococcus* spp., *Streptococcus* spp., *Enterococcus* spp., *Enterobacteriaceae* spp., *Proteus* spp., *Klebsiella* spp., *Pseudomonas* spp., *Bacteroides* spp.

Mild (Treatment duration: 7–14 days)

- ▨ Cephalexin 500 mg PO four times daily
- ▨ If MRSA suspected:
  - – **ADD** doxycycline 100 mg PO two times daily **OR**
  - – TMP/SMX (DS) 1–2 tablets PO two times daily
- ▨ If severe PCN allergy:
  - – Clindamycin 450 mg PO three times daily

Moderate (Treatment duration: 7–21 days)

- ▨ Ceftriaxone 1 g IV daily (consider 2 g if > 100 kg or severe infection)
- ▨ Ampicillin/sulbactam 3 g IV four times daily
- ▨ If MRSA suspected **ADD:**
  - – Vancomycin 25–30 mg/kg IV loading dose **THEN** 15–20 mg/kg IV two–three times daily **OR**
  - – Doxycycline 100 mg PO/IV two times daily **OR**
  - – TMP/SMX (DS) 1–2 tablets PO two times daily
- ▨ If severe PCN allergy:
  - – Clindamycin 450 mg PO or 600 mg IV three times daily **AND** levofloxacin 750 mg PO/IV once daily

Severe (Treatment duration: 14–28 days)

- ▨ Vancomycin 25–30 mg/kg IV loading dose **THEN** 15–20 mg/kg IV two–three times daily **AND** metronidazole 500 mg IV three times daily **PLUS:**
  - – Cefepime 2 g IV two–three times daily **OR**
  - – Ciprofloxacin 400 mg IV three times daily **OR**
  - – Levofloxacin 750 mg IV daily **OR**
  - – Aztreonam 2 g IV three times daily

SKIN & SOFT TISSUE

PEARLS

- Osteomyelitis should be considered in all cases of deep ulceration. Ulcers with evidence of infection and a positive probe-to-bone test are likely to be complicated by osteomyelitis
- Plain radiographs may show foreign bodies, soft-tissue gas, or bony abnormalities, but have poor sensitivity and specificity for osteomyelitis (MRI with gadolinium is the imaging modality of choice)
- Cultures should be obtained from cleaned and debrided wounds; tissue cultures are preferred
- Most diabetic ulcers are polymicrobial, with staphylococci the most common causative organism

FELON

Common organisms: *S. aureus*, *Streptococcus* spp.
(Treatment is I&D and 7–10 days of antibiotic therapy)
- Cephalexin 500 mg PO four times daily **PLUS:**
  - TMP/SMX (DS) 1–2 tablets PO two times daily **OR**
  - Doxycycline 100 mg PO two times daily **OR**
  - Clindamycin 450 mg PO three times daily

PEARLS

- Vesicles are consistent with herpetic infection (do not I&D), consider topical acyclovir 5%
- Consider local MRSA resistance patterns
- *Eikenella corrodens* should be considered if felon is a result of nail biting or patient immunosuppressed, consider **ADDING**
  - Amoxicillin/clavulanate 875 mg PO two times daily
- Did you know the current POTUS is from Delaware?

FOLLICULITIS

Common organisms: *S. aureus*, *Pseudomonas* spp.

Usually self-resolving in 1-2 weeks. If no resolution consider:
Topical Treatment
- Topical clindamycin 1% to affected area two times daily as needed
- Mupirocin 2% ointment to affected area three times daily as needed
- Topical erythromycin 2% to affected area two times daily as needed
- Chlorhexidine containing antiseptic cleanser daily for 1–2 weeks

PEARLS

- Treatment for hot tub folliculitis generally not indicated but may consider chlorhexidine cleanser

IMPETIGO

Common organisms: *S. aureus* (*MSSA* and *CA-MRSA*) and Group A *Streptococcus*

- Isolated lesions
  - Mupirocin 2% ointment three times daily for 5 days
- Numerous lesions
  - Cephalexin 250 mg (Ⓟ 6.25-12.5 mg/kg) PO four times daily for 7 days
- If MRSA suspected:
  - TMP/SMX (DS) 1–2 tablets (Ⓟ 4–6 mg/kg) PO two times daily for 7 days
  - Doxycycline 100 mg PO two times daily for 7 days
  - Clindamycin 450 mg (Ⓟ 10 mg/kg) PO three times daily for 7 days

PEARLS

- Topical and oral antibiotics are equally effective for treating cases of bullous and nonbullous impetigo with a limited number of lesions
- Consider oral antibiotics for cases with multiple lesions or in outbreaks affecting multiple people

MASTITIS

Common organisms: *S. aureus, Streptococcus* spp., *E. coli*
(Treatment duration: 10–14 days)

- Cephalexin 500 mg PO four times daily
- Amoxicillin/clavulanate 875 mg PO two times daily
- If severe PCN allergy:
  - Clindamycin 450 mg PO three times daily (questionable safety if breastfeeding)
- If MRSA suspected:
  - Clindamycin 450 mg PO three times daily (questionable safety if breastfeeding
  - TMP/SMX (DS) 1 tablet PO two times daily (consider adding strep coverage; questionable safety if breastfeeding)
  - If severe infection: vancomycin 15–20 mg/kg IV two–three times daily

PEARLS

- Symptomatic treatment: warm compress prior to breastfeeding, cold compresses after breastfeeding, hydration, bed rest, ibuprofen, increased frequency of breastfeeding/pumping, optimizing breastfeeding technique

SKIN & SOFT TISSUE

NECROTIZING FASCIITIS (INCLUDING FOURNIER'S GANGRENE, GAS GANGRENE)

Common organisms: *Streptococcus* spp., *Bacteroides* spp., *Staphylococcus* spp., *Clostridioides* spp., *Enterococcus* spp.

- Vancomycin 25–30 mg/kg IV loading dose **THEN** 15–20 mg/kg IV two–three times daily **PLUS:**
  - Cefepime 2 g IV two–three times daily **AND** metronidazole 500 mg IV three times daily **OR**
  - Piperacillin/tazobactam 4.5 g IV four times daily **OR**
  - Imipenem/cilastatin 1 g IV three times daily
- If severe PCN allergy:
  - Vancomycin 25-30 mg/kg IV loading dose **THEN** 15-20 mg/kg IV two-three times daily **AND** metronidazole 500 mg IV four times daily **AND** levofloxacin 750 mg IV once daily
- In consultation with ID, consider adding clindamycin 600-900 mg IV three times daily for toxin suppression

PEARLS

- Prompt surgical evaluation is critical
- CT helps define extent of disease, may identify source but should not delay surgical involvement
- Subcutaneous gas is highly specific, but not sensitive, for necrotizing fasciitis
- Fournier's is usually polymicrobial; *Pseudomonas* and *Staphylococcus* are often present
- Consider replacing metronidazole with clindamycin to inhibit toxin production in cases where Group A *Streptococcus* is suspected or confirmed via culture

PARONYCHIA

Common organisms: *Staphylococcus* spp., *Streptococcus* spp., *Candida* spp.

- I&D is the treatment of choice
- If there is no drainable abscess and only inflammation present, warm compresses may aid in spontaneous drainage
- Reserve antibiotics for associated cellulitis

SKIN & SOFT TISSUE

TINEA

Tinea Capitis

Common organisms: *Microsporum canis*, *Trichophyton* spp.

Use one topical treatment **AND** one systemic medication

- ▣ Topical
  - – Ketoconazole 2% shampoo three times weekly for 2 weeks (age ≥ 12 years old)
  - – Selenium sulfide 2.25% shampoo three times weekly for 2 weeks

AND

- ▣ Systemic
  - – Itraconazole 200 mg ((P) 5 mg/kg) PO once daily for 2–4 weeks
  - – Griseofulvin 500 mg ((P) 10 mg/kg ultramicrosize, 20 mg/kg microsize, 20 mg/kg suspension) PO once daily for 12 weeks
  - – Terbinafine 250 mg ((P) 62.5 mg if < 20 kg, 125 mg if 20–40 kg, 250 mg if > 40 kg) PO daily for 4–6 weeks if suspected *Trichophyton* infection

Tinea Corporis, Cruris, Pedis, or Manuum

Common organisms: *Trichophyton* spp., *Epidermophyton floccosum*

- ▣ Isolated or mild/moderate severity
  - – Topical clotrimazole 1% or ketoconazole 2% two times daily for 4 weeks (or for 1 week after lesions have healed)
- ▣ Severe, bullous, or extensive disease
  - – Fluconazole 150 mg ((P) 6 mg/kg) PO once weekly for 2–4 weeks
  - – Itraconazole 200 mg ((P) 5 mg/kg) PO once daily (two times daily for pedis/manuum) for 1 week
  - – Griseofulvin 500 mg–1 g ((P) 10 mg/kg ultramicrosize, 20 mg/kg microsize) PO once daily for 2–4 weeks
  - – Terbinafine 250 mg ((P) 125 mg if < 25 kg, 187.5 mg if 25–35 kg, 250 mg if > 35 kg) PO daily for 1–2 weeks

Tinea Versicolor (Pityriasis Versicolor)

Common organisms: *Malassezia furfur*, *Pityrosporum orbiculare*

- ▣ Topical
  - – Ketoconazole 2% cream once daily for 10–21 days (age ≥ 12 years old)
  - – Ketoconazole 2% shampoo once (age ≥ 12 years old)
  - – Terbinafine 1% solution once daily for 7 days (age ≥ 12 years old)
  - – Ciclopirox 1% cream twice daily for 14 days (age ≥ 10 years old)
  - – Selenium sulfide 2.5% lotion, apply for 10 min on skin daily for 1 week
  - – Zinc pyrithione 1% shampoo, apply for 10 min on skin daily for 1 week

SKIN & SOFT TISSUE

- Systemic
  - Fluconazole 300 mg (ⓟ 12 mg/kg) PO once weekly for 2 weeks
  - Itraconazole 200 mg (ⓟ 5 mg/kg) PO once daily for 5–7 days

PEARLS

- Systemic antifungals are associated with hepatic injury
- Systemic antifungals are typically not approved for pediatric use, though documented use has indicated similar safety and efficacy as for adults
- Itraconazole is associated with heart failure, and dysrhythmias have resulted from drug-drug interactions. Not recommended for patients with ventricular dysfunction or CHF
- Advise griseofulvin to be administered with fatty foods to improve absorption
- Griseofulvin may decrease the efficacy of oral contraceptives
- In cases of kerion formation, oral steroids may help reduce the risk of permanent hair loss
- Pigment changes typically take several weeks to resolve after successful treatment of tinea versicolor

VARICELLA (CHICKENPOX) OR ZOSTER (SHINGLES)

Note: Acyclovir dosing based on ideal body weight

Pediatric

- Immunocompetent and age < 12 years
  - Supportive care, such as frequent bathing, calamine lotion, and acetaminophen for fever (ibuprofen may be associated with life-threatening skin infections)
- At risk for complicated disease (age > 12 years, cardiopulmonary disease, chronic steroid therapy, etc.)
  - Acyclovir 20 mg/kg PO four times daily for 5 days
- Immunocompromised
  - Acyclovir 10 mg/kg IV three times daily for 7–10 days

Adult

- Immunocompetent
  - Acyclovir 800 mg PO five times daily for 7–10 days
  - Valacyclovir 1 g PO three times daily for 7 days
  - Famciclovir 500 mg PO three times daily for 7 days
- Immunocompromised
  - Acyclovir 10 mg/kg IV three times daily for 10 days

SKIN & SOFT TISSUE

PEARLS

- Herpes zoster ophthalmicus: Recommend consultation with Ophthalmology
- Herpes zoster oticus (vesicles in auditory canal, possibly part of triad of Ramsay Hunt syndrome with ipsilateral ear pain and facial nerve paralysis): consider **ADDING** prednisone after otolaryngology consultation
- Infected individuals should keep rash covered (until crusted), perform hand hygiene frequently, and avoid contact with immunocompromised individuals, premature or low birth weight infants, and individuals who are pregnant
- Consider admission of pregnant patients with varicella
- Complications include encephalitis, pneumonia, and hepatitis
- Treatment should begin within 24 hrs of the varicella rash or 72 hrs from zoster symptom onset due to the potential decrease in efficacy as time wanes, unless there is still vesicular eruption

SKIN & SOFT TISSUE

ANTHRAX

Anthrax is a reportable disease. In any case of suspected bioterrorism, contact your local health department and the CDC Emergency Operations Center at 770-488-7100

Common organism: *Bacillus anthracis*
Post-exposure Prophylaxis or Cutaneous Anthrax
(Treatment duration: 60 days; 7–10 days if agricultural exposure and no inhalation)

- Doxycycline 100 mg (🅟 2.2 mg/kg) PO two times daily
- Ciprofloxacin 500 mg (🅟 15 mg/kg) PO two times daily
- Levofloxacin 750 mg PO daily (🅟 < 50 kg: 8 mg/kg PO two times daily, max 250 mg/dose)
- Clindamycin 600 mg (🅟 10 mg/kg) PO three times daily
- If PCN susceptible strain:
  - Amoxicillin 1 g (🅟 25 mg/kg) PO three times daily
  - Penicillin VK 500 mg (🅟 15 mg/kg) PO four times daily

Systemic Anthrax
(Treatment duration: at least 2 weeks, **THEN** convert to post-exposure prophylaxis if inhalation exposure)

- If meningitis suspected/confirmed:
  - Ciprofloxacin 400 mg (🅟 10 mg/kg) IV three times daily **AND** meropenem 2 g (🅟 40 mg/kg) IV three times daily **AND** linezolid 600 mg two times daily (🅟 age < 12 years 10 mg/kg three times daily, max 600 mg/dose) IV
    - Consider dexamethasone 10 mg (🅟 0.15 mg/kg up to 10 mg) IV four times daily
- If meningitis has been ruled out:
  - Ciprofloxacin 400 mg (🅟 10 mg/kg) IV three times daily **OR** meropenem 2 g (🅟 20 mg/kg) IV three times daily **OR** linezolid 600 mg two times daily (🅟 age < 12 yrs, 10 mg/kg three times daily, max 600 mg/dose) IV **OR** (second-line) doxycycline 100 mg (🅟 2.2 mg/kg) IV two times daily

PEARLS

- CDC guidance is recommended for all cases of anthrax
- Isolation precautions
  - Bioterrorism/spore-containing powder exposure: full decontamination, protective clothing/gown and use of N95 or powered air-purifying respirator (PAPR)
  - Agricultural exposure (grazing farm animals, soil): human to human transmission typically does not occur, standard PPE recommended

BIOTERRORISM

- – Contact precautions for large draining lesions
- ▣ Anthrax vaccine on days 0, 14, and 28 for postexposure prophylaxis in addition to antibiotics
- ▣ Vaccination status does not alter treatment recommendations
- ▣ Consider antitoxin therapy (raxibacumab or Anthrax Immune Globulin) in consultation with the CDC
- ▣ Inhalational
  - – **Prodrome period:** begins as flu-like syndrome for 2–3 days; prominent symptoms of cough and chest discomfort help distinguish from flu
  - – **Acute phase:** sudden onset of hypoxia, dyspnea, shock, signs of hemorrhagic mediastinitis, hemorrhagic meningitis
  - – Gastrointestinal and oropharyngeal anthrax should be treated as inhalational
- ▣ Cutaneous
  - – Nontender skin lesion with surrounding edema and lymphadenopathy
  - – Evolves from papule to vesicle to burst vesicle with central black eschar over the course of a week

BOTULISM

In any case of suspected bioterrorism, contact your local health department and the CDC Emergency Operations Center at 770-488-7100

Common organism: *Clostridioides* spp.

Foodborne Botulism

- ▣ Equine Serum Heptavalent Botulism Antitoxin for patients > 1 year old
- ▣ For antitoxin, contact local and state health departments. If not available, contact the CDC
- ▣ Skin test for sensitivity prior to administering antitoxin and monitor for anaphylaxis during infusion
- ▣ Dose is one vial for adults > 17 years old. See package insert for specific administration instructions and pediatric dosing chart

Infant Botulism

- ▣ Human botulinum antitoxin (BabyBIG) for infants < 1 year is only available through California Dept. of Health, Infant Botulism Program: 510-231-7600

Inhalational Botulism

- ▣ For suspected inhalation botulism, immediately contact the CDC
- ▣ Same treatment as foodborne botulism
- ▣ Inhalational botulism does not occur naturally; suspect bioterrorism

Wound Botulism
▪ Antitoxin, surgical debridement, and antibiotics; see Necrotizing Fasciitis, p. 68

PEARLS
▪ State public health department and/or CDC guidance is recommended for all cases of botulism
▪ **Isolation precautions:** No human-to-human transmission, so isolation not required
▪ **Adult Dx:** (1) symmetric, descending flaccid paralysis with bulbar palsies (4D's: **D**iplopia, **D**ysarthria, **D**ysphonia, **D**ysphagia), (2) afebrile patient, (3) clear sensorium, (4) no sensory deficits except blurred vision (consider other Dx if sensory deficit)
▪ **Infant Dx:** constipation often first but can be overlooked, most often present with poor feeding, ptosis, lethargy, and hypotonia
▪ Foodborne botulism diagnosis obtained by serum assay for toxin
▪ Infant botulism diagnosis is obtained by stool direct toxin analysis and culture for organism
▪ Antibiotics **NOT** routinely required for foodborne, inhalational, or infant botulism

SMALLPOX

In any case of suspected bioterrorism, contact your local health department and the CDC Emergency Operations Center at 770-488-7100.

Postexposure Prophylaxis
▪ Vaccinia virus vaccine (within 3 days of exposure)
  — Obtain from State Health Department or the CDC

Active Disease
▪ Vaccination within 3 days can prevent or reduce severity of disease
▪ Vaccination within 7 days may modify disease course
▪ Provide adequate fluid intake, pain and fever relief, and possible antibiotics for bacterial superinfection from open lesions
▪ Tecovirimat and brincidofovir are oral agents FDA-approved for the treatment of smallpox; there have been no trials in humans

PEARLS
▪ CDC guidance is recommended for all cases of smallpox
▪ Isolation precautions
  — Airborne and contact transmissibility
  — Isolation in negative pressure
▪ If directly exposed to smallpox, there are no contraindications for postexposure vaccination in an emergent setting

BIOTERRORISM

- Prodromal illness may include fever and malaise, followed by centrifugal maculopapular rash on skin (including palms, soles, and mucosa)
- Often confused with Varicella (chickenpox), which manifests as lesions that are in various stages and excludes palms and soles

TULAREMIA

In any case of suspected bioterrorism, contact your local health department and the CDC Emergency Operations Center at 770-488-7100

Common organism: *Francisella tularensis*, a gram-negative coccobacillus

Post-exposure Prophylaxis or Mass Casualty
(Treatment duration: 10 days)
- Doxycycline 100 mg (Ⓟ 2.2 mg/kg daily, max 200 mg/day) PO two times daily for at least 14 days
- Ciprofloxacin 500 mg (Ⓟ 15 mg/kg, max 1 g/day) PO two times daily for at least 10 days

Active Disease or Contained Casualty, Preferred
(Treatment duration: 10 days)
- Streptomycin 1 g (Ⓟ 15 mg/kg, max 2 g/day) IM two times daily
- Gentamicin 5 mg/kg IV/IM once daily (Ⓟ 2.5 mg/kg IV/IM three times daily) (*see weight-based dosing, p. 101*)
- If meningitis suspected: **ADD** chloramphenicol 15 mg/kg (Ⓟ 15 mg/kg, max 4 g/day) IV four times daily for 14–21 days

Alternatives (mild-moderate symptoms, active disease)
- Ciprofloxacin 400 mg (Ⓟ 15 mg/kg, max 1 g/day) IV two times daily for 10–14 days
- Doxycycline 100 mg (Ⓟ 2.2 mg/kg, max 200 mg/day) IV two times daily for 14–21 days

PEARLS
- CDC guidance is recommended for all cases of tularemia
- Isolation precautions: No human-to-human transmission, so isolation not required
- Transmission vectors: ticks, flies, rabbits, contaminated aerosols, dusts, and water
- **Pneumonic:** (most serious form) flu-like symptoms, nonproductive cough, and respiratory distress
- **Ulceroglandular:** (most common form) local papule evolving to an ulcer, regional lymphadenopathy, fever, and flu-like symptoms
- **Typhoidal:** Generalized symptoms including fever, headache, abdominal pain, nausea, vomiting, and diarrhea
- Rabbits can give birth to up to 14 babies—called kittens—in a single litter

BIOTERRORISM

YERSINIA

In any case of suspected bioterrorism, contact your local health department and the CDC Emergency Operations Center at 770-488-7100

Common organism: *Yersinia pestis*

Post-exposure Prophylaxis

(Treatment duration: 7 days)

- Doxycycline 100 mg (Ⓟ 2.2 mg/kg) PO two times daily
- Ciprofloxacin 500 mg (Ⓟ 15 mg/kg) PO two times daily

Active Disease

(Treatment duration: 10–14 days)

- Ciprofloxacin 750 mg (Ⓟ 15 mg/kg) PO two times daily
- Ciprofloxacin 400 mg (Ⓟ 10 mg/kg) IV three times daily
- Levofloxacin 750 mg PO/IV once daily (Ⓟ 8 mg/kg PO two times daily, max 250 mg/dose)
- Moxifloxacin 400 mg PO/IV once daily
- Gentamicin 5 mg/kg IV/IM once daily (Ⓟ 4.5-7.5 mg/kg IV/IM once daily)
- Streptomycin 1 g (Ⓟ 15 mg/kg, max 1 g/dose) IV/IM two times daily
- Doxycycline 200 mg loading dose, **THEN** 100 mg (Ⓟ 4.4 mg/kg loading dose, **THEN** 2.2 mg/kg) PO/IV two times daily

PEARLS

- CDC guidance is recommended for all cases of yersinia
- Start treatment if suggestive clinical signs and exposure history, do not wait for diagnostic test results
- Isolation precautions
  - Respiratory transmissibility in pneumonic form (droplet precautions)
  - Contact transmissibility in bubonic form
- Transmission vector is the flea
- Streptomycin and chloramphenicol are not widely available in the U.S.
- In pregnancy, treat with gentamicin **PLUS** ciprofloxacin **OR** levofloxacin, doxycycline, or ciprofloxacin at the standard adult dose
- **Bubonic (most common):** Tender, painful, swollen lymph nodes (buboes) with fever, headache, and chills
- **Pneumonic:** Rapidly progressive flu-like illness with bloody sputum, respiratory failure, and shock
- **Septicemic:** Fever, chills, weakness, shock, DIC, purpuric skin lesions, and gangrene

RABIES

Post-exposure prophylaxis, without prior vaccination

- Rabies immune globulin (RIG): 20 IU/kg (infiltrate as much as possible subcutaneously at wound site, inject remainder into deltoid IM) on day 0
- Rabies vaccine: 1 mL deltoid IM on days 0, 3, 7, 14
- Immunosuppressed patients require additional rabies vaccine 1 mL deltoid IM on day 28

Note: Immune globulin and vaccine must be given at separate sites

Post-exposure prophylaxis, with prior vaccination and documented antibody response to prior vaccination

- Rabies vaccine: 1 mL deltoid IM on days 0 and 3

PEARLS

- Rabies vaccines and RIG are safe and effective in pregnant and lactating women
- Avoid corticosteroids, antimalarials, and other immunosuppressive agents during post-exposure therapy as they may prevent immunity; immunosuppressed individuals may need antibody titers checked and may require management by PCP/public health
- Wound should be extensively cleaned with soap and water
- If the calculated dose of RIG is insufficient to infiltrate all wounds, sterile saline may be used to dilute it 2- to 3-fold to permit thorough infiltration
- Recommended site for IM administration is the deltoid area for adults and children age ≥ 2 years, and the anterolateral area of the thigh for children age < 2 years
- Update tetanus immunization if indicated
- Saliva or brain/nervous system tissue are the only body contents of an infected mammal that transmit disease
- Domestic mammals (eg, dogs, cats, ferrets): If the animal can be observed for 10 days and is asymptomatic, treatment not necessary
- Wild carnivores (eg, skunks, raccoons, foxes, coyotes): Consider rabid and begin therapy
- Bat exposure: Post-exposure prophylaxis should be administered for both bite and non-bite exposures
- Livestock, rodents (eg, hamsters, rats, mice, gerbils, squirrels, chipmunks, rabbits): Rarely carry the disease and treatment usually not necessary

ENVIRONMENTAL EXPOSURES

TETANUS

Active Disease

- Administer immunoglobulin prior to surgical debridement
- Human tetanus immune globulin (TIG) 500 international units IM with partial administration around identified wounds **PLUS:**
  - Metronidazole 500 mg (P 10 mg/kg) IV three times daily **OR**
  - Penicillin G 4 million units (P 25,000–50,000 IU/kg) IV four times daily
- If TIG is unavailable: intravenous immunoglobulin (IVIG) 200–400 mg/kg IV
- If indicated, administer Tdap vaccination in opposite extremity from TIG

Prophylaxis

- If > 5 yrs since last booster in tetanus-prone wound or > 10 years in any wound:
  - Tetanus/diphtheria/acellular pertussis (Tdap) vaccine 0.5 mL IM
- If < 3 doses of primary vaccination series **OR** status is unknown **OR** patient has HIV or other immunocompromised state **AND** wound is tetanus-prone:
  - Human tetanus immune globulin (TIG) 250 units IM **AND** tetanus/diphtheria/acellular pertussis (Tdap) vaccine 0.5 mL IM
    - Administer Tdap vaccination in opposite extremity from TIG

PEARLS

- Tetanus is a clinical diagnosis and may present without wound. Suspect if history of tetanus prone injury and inadequate immunization. No definitive laboratory test exists
- High-risk patients for inadequate vaccination include IVDU, immigrants, rural patients, and the elderly
- Incubation period can be 3–21 days (average 10 days); neonatal tetanus (typically from infected umbilical stump) typically seen 4–14 days from birth
- Primary treatments are muscle relaxation (first-line benzodiazepines, second-line neuromuscular blocking agents) and airway management
- Wide debridement of wound in active disease is a critical aspect of therapy to prevent further germination of spores

ENVIRONMENTAL EXPOSURES

CRYPTOCOCCUS NEOFORMANS

Pulmonary (Mild to Moderate Disease)
- ▣ Fluconazole 400-800 mg PO once daily for up to 6 months
  - – Consult ID for specific dosing and duration, per patient-specific factors

Meningitis, Disseminated, or Severe Pulmonary Disease
- ▣ Liposomal amphotericin B 3-4 mg/kg IV daily **AND** flucytosine 25 mg/kg PO four times daily for 2 weeks **THEN** fluconazole 400-800 mg PO once daily for 8 weeks

PEARLS
- ▣ Amphotericin B is associated with drug fevers, rigors, renal insufficiency, electrolyte disturbances, and anemia
- ▣ Consider fluids, acetaminophen, and diphenhydramine at time of infusion of amphotericin B to decrease drug infusion reactions and renal insufficiency
- ▣ Serial LP may be therapeutic for increased ICP

FEBRILE NEUTROPENIA

Common organisms: *Staphylococcus* spp., *Streptococcus* spp., *Enterococcus* spp., *Corynebacterium* spp., *E. coli*, *Klebsiella* spp., *Pseudomonas* spp.

Low-risk Outpatient
- ▣ Ciprofloxacin 750 mg PO two times daily **PLUS:**
  - – Amoxicillin/clavulanate 875 mg PO two times daily **OR**
  - – If severe PCN allergy:
    - • **REPLACE** amoxicillin/clavulanate with clindamycin 450-600 mg PO three times daily
- ▣ Levofloxacin 750 mg PO once daily

Inpatient
- ▣ Cefepime 2 g IV three times daily
- ▣ Piperacillin/tazobactam 4.5 g IV four times daily
- ▣ Imipenem/cilastatin 1 g IV three times daily
- ▣ Meropenem 1 g IV three times daily

Criteria for including vancomycin
- ▣ Catheter-related infection, PNA, skin/soft tissue infection, or hypotension/shock

IMMUNE-COMPROMISED HOST INFECTIONS

- ▪ Known colonization with MRSA or multi-drug resistant *Streptococcus*
- ▪ Cultures showing gram-positive organism with unknown susceptibility

If severe PCN allergy:
- ▪ Meropenem 1 g IV three times daily **OR**
- ▪ Aztreonam 2 g IV three times daily **AND** vancomycin 25–30 mg/kg IV loading dose **THEN** 15–20 mg/kg IV two–three times daily

PEARLS
- ▪ Neutropenia is defined as ANC (absolute neutrophil count) < 500 cells/mm^3 or when a drop to this level is anticipated in the next 48 hrs and signifies higher risk (WBC nadir 7–14 days after chemotherapy)
- ▪ **MASCC (Multinational Association for Supportive Care in Cancer)**: risk stratification tool that can be used to identify patients appropriate for outpatient management. Should be done in consultation with oncologist
- ▪ Antifungal therapy is not indicated in the ED unless there is a known fungal infection
- ▪ Antiviral therapy is generally not recommended for empiric therapy. In influenza outbreak or exposure, flu-like symptoms should prompt treatment with neuraminidase inhibitors

PNEUMOCYSTIS JIROVECI PNEUMONIA (PCP)

Mild
(Treatment duration: 21 days)
- ▪ TMP/SMX (DS) 2 tablets PO three times daily
- ▪ Dapsone 100 mg PO once daily **AND** TMP 5 mg/kg PO three times daily
- ▪ Atovaquone 750 mg PO two times daily with food
- ▪ Primaquine 30 mg PO once daily **AND** clindamycin 450 mg PO three times daily

Moderate/Severe
(Treatment duration: 21 days)
- ▪ TMP/SMX 5 mg/kg IV three-four times daily
- ▪ Primaquine 30 mg PO once daily **AND** clindamycin 900 mg IV three times daily (ⓟ 450 mg PO four times daily)
- ▪ Pentamidine 4 mg/kg IV once daily over 60 min

Pregnant
- ▪ TMP/SMX as above **AND** IF in the first trimester **ADD** folic acid 0.4 mg PO/IV once daily to decrease risk of birth defects

PEARLS

- Corticosteroids are indicated for moderate to severe cases (including pregnancy) which is defined as: PaO2 < 70 mmHg or A-a gradient > 35 mmHg. Initiate prednisone taper:
  - **Days 1–5:** 40 mg PO two times daily
  - **Days 6–10:** 40 mg PO once daily
  - **Days 11–21:** 20 mg PO once daily
- Dapsone and primaquine may cause methemoglobinemia and/or hemolysis
- If patient is on TMP/SMX prophylaxis and develops PCP, standard dose TMP/SMX is still considered first line

TOXOPLASMOSIS

Common organism: *Toxoplasmosis gondii*
Note: Patients who are immunocompetent and not pregnant usually do not require treatment unless symptoms are severe or prolonged

(Treatment duration: 4–6 weeks)

- Pyrimethamine 200 mg PO once, **THEN** 50 mg (pt weight < 60 kg) to 75 mg (pt weight > 60 kg) PO once daily **AND** leucovorin 10–25 mg PO once daily **PLUS:**
  - Sulfadiazine 1 g (< 60 kg) to 1.5 g (> 60 kg) PO four times daily **OR**
  - Clindamycin 600 mg PO/IV four times daily **OR**
  - Azithromycin 1200 mg PO once daily **OR**
  - Atovaquone 1500 mg PO two times daily
- TMP/SMX 5 mg/kg PO/IV two times daily

PEARLS

- Preferred treatment is pyrimethamine; however, there is limited availability in the U.S. through special pharmacy programs
- If severe sulfa allergy, patients should be referred for desensitization
- Leucovorin (ie, folinic acid) should be administered concomitantly to prevent bone marrow suppression
- Consult OB in pregnant patients
- Treatment duration is 12 months for infants with congenital toxoplasmosis and HIV
- Serious complications include encephalitis, pneumonitis, chorioretinitis, and myocarditis

IMMUNE-COMPROMISED HOST INFECTIONS

HIV AND HEPATITIS

Evaluate the Exposed Person and the Source

- ▫ Wash wounds and skin with soap and water. Flush mucous membranes with water
- ▫ Determine HCV, HBV, and HIV status of source. Perform Rapid HIV test when possible
- ▫ Assess immune status of exposed person for HBV infection (ie, by history of hepatitis B vaccination and vaccine response). Vaccine response should be tested if not previously determined (Anti–HBs)
- ▫ Consider baseline labs per local PEP protocol
- ▫ Note that feces, sweat, saliva, vomitus, and urine are NOT considered infectious bodily fluids unless contaminated by blood

Provide Information to the Exposed Person

- ▫ Risk of developing serologic evidence of HBV via percutaneous exposure, if unvaccinated
  - – Risk = 23–37% if blood source is HBsAg (+) and HBeAg (–)
  - – Risk = 37–62% if HBsAg (+) and HBeAg (+)
- ▫ Multiple doses of HBIG combined with HBV vaccine series given within 1 week of exposure confer approximately 75% protection from a percutaneous injury with exposure to HBsAg (+) blood
- ▫ Risk of transmission of HCV from HCV+ source is approximately 1.8%
- ▫ Risk of transmission of HIV from HIV+ source
  - – Percutaneous exposure: 0.3%
  - – Mucous membrane exposure: 0.09%
  - – Injuries with hollow-bore needle or from sources with high viral load are higher risk

Give PEP for Exposure Posing Risk of Infectious Transmission

- ▫ Initiate PEP as soon as possible, preferably within 2 hrs of exposure
- ▫ Treatment presumed ineffective if started > 72 hrs after exposure for HIV
- ▫ When HBIG or hepatitis B vaccine indicated, administer ASAP, preferably within 24 hrs
- ▫ Offer pregnancy testing to all women of child-bearing age

Hepatitis B Virus

- ▫ Treatment depends on previous vaccination history and immunity of the exposed person as well as HBV status of the source
  - – If HBV status of source is unobtainable, estimate risk of transmission based on epidemiologic factors such as local prevalence
  - – If exposed person is unvaccinated, administer HBV vaccine series
  - – If source is HBsAg(+), unvaccinated exposed person should receive HBV vaccine series and HBIG
  - – If exposed person is vaccinated, check baseline labs (HBsAg, anti-HBs, total anti-HBc) or if no labs drawn, administer single booster HBV vaccine dose

Recommended Hepatitis B Virus Post-exposure Prophylaxis

	Source HBsAg (+)	Source HBsAg (−)	Source unknown or not available for testing
Unvaccinated	HBIG X 1 and initiate HBV vaccine series*	Initiate HBV vaccine series	HBIG x 1 **AND** initiate HBV vaccine series
Previously vaccinated, responder (anti-HBs > 10 mIU/mL)	No treatment	No treatment	No treatment
Previously vaccinated, one series, nonresponder (anti-HBs < 10 mIU/mL)	HBIG X 1 and initiate revaccination*	No treatment	If known high-risk source, treat as if source were HBsAg (+)
Previously vaccinated, two series, nonresponder (anti-HBs < 10 mIU/mL)	HBIG X 2	No treatment	If known high-risk source, treat as if source were HBsAg (+)

*Administer at two separate sites

Treatment Dosing

- Hepatitis B Immune Globulin (HBIG) 0.06 mL/kg IM
- Vaccination series: HBV vaccine (Engerix-B 20 mcg or Recombivax HB 10 mcg) administered IM at 0, 1 month, and 6 months
- Pregnancy or lactation is not a contraindication to vaccination

Hepatitis C Virus

- For known exposures to Hepatitis C, perform baseline anti-HCV and ALT on exposed person and obtain baseline testing for anti-HCV from source
- Perform follow-up testing with HCV RNA by PCR in 3–6 weeks after exposure **AND** with anti-HCV 4–6 *months* after exposure
  - If positive, refer to HCV specialist for supplemental anti-HCV testing and treatment
- No drug regimen is currently proven beneficial for prophylactic treatment

(P) = Pediatric dosing

HIV

- HIV PEP is time-sensitive and should be given ASAP (< 72 hrs of exposure), without waiting for source testing unless rapid test will result within 2 hrs
- PEP is generally not warranted if source HIV status is unknown, but should be considered if exposure source has HIV risk factors

Recommended HIV Post-Exposure Prophylaxis

- Three-drug regimens are now recommended for all HIV exposures
- PEP is given for 28 days, but may be discontinued if source tests negative for HIV

Preferred Three-Drug Regimen for HIV PEP

- Raltegravir 400 mg PO two times daily **AND** tenofovir DF 300 mg PO once daily **AND** emtricitabine 200 mg PO once daily (combination tablet available)
  - If CrCl is 30–49 mL/min, **THEN** decrease frequency to every other day (other regimens exist; consult ID)
- Alternative regimens (eg, dolutegravir once daily) may be available with expert consultation
- Test CBC, renal, and hepatic function at baseline and 2 weeks after starting PEP regimen
- HIV-antibody testing should be performed at baseline, 6 weeks, 12 weeks, and 6 months

Resources for Consultation

- Clinician Consultation Center PEPline: 888-448-4911 or http://nccc.ucsf.edu/clinical-resources/pep-resources
- HIV Antiretroviral Pregnancy Registry: 800-258-4263 or www.apregistry.com
- U.S. Department of Health and Human Services AIDS info: https://aidsinfo.nih.gov
- Database of antiretroviral drug interactions: http://chi.ucsf.edu

LICE—HEAD/BODY/PUBIC

OTC

- ▪ Permethrin 1% lotion or shampoo (first-line) — apply to clean and damp hair, rinse after 10 min, **THEN** repeat in 9 days (> 2 months old)
- ▪ Pyrethrin 0.3% + piperonyl butoxide 0.4% shampoo/mousse — apply to dry hair, rinse after 10 min, **THEN** repeat in 9 days (> 2 years old)

Rx

- ▪ **Head**
  - — Spinosad 0.9% topical suspension — apply to dry hair, rinse with warm water after 10 min, may repeat in 7 days (> 6 months old)
  - — Benzyl alcohol 5% lotion — apply to dry hair, rinse with cool water after 10 min, **THEN** repeat in 7 days (> 6 months old)
  - — Ivermectin 0.5% lotion — apply to dry hair, rinse with warm water after 10 min (> 6 months old)
  - — Ivermectin 200 mcg/kg PO once **THEN** repeat on day 10 (caution in pregnant/breastfeeding women and in children < 15 kg)
- ▪ **Body/Pubic**
  - — Permethrin 5% cream — apply to entire clean body from neck down (include head/neck in infants and children), wash off after 8–12 hrs; may repeat in 2 weeks (> 2 months old)
  - — Ivermectin 200–400 mcg/kg PO once (consider if topical therapy fails)

PEARLS

- ▪ All members of the household should be examined
- ▪ Do not use conditioner before using lice medication, and do not wash hair for 1–2 days after medication has been removed
- ▪ Use in conjunction with wet combing
- ▪ For children < 2 years old, wet combing is a reasonable alternative to medical therapy
- ▪ Children may finish the school day and return to school after the first application of treatment
- ▪ For eyelash infestation, apply ophthalmic-grade petroleum jelly two times daily for 10 days
- ▪ Screen for other STDs/STIs in patients with pubic lice; abstain from sexual contact until infestation clears
- ▪ Wash clothing, towels, and bedding in hot water; fumigant sprays are not needed and may be harmful
- ▪ For resistant cases, consider oral ivermectin
- ▪ Patients may develop secondary cellulitis due to extensive excoriations

PEDIATRIC INFECTIONS

PINWORMS

Common organism: *Enterobius vermicularis*
- Albendazole 400 mg (℗ 200 mg in children < 20 kg) PO once, **THEN** repeat in 2 weeks
- Mebendazole 100 mg PO once, **THEN** repeat in 2 weeks
- Pyrantel pamoate 11 mg/kg PO once (℗ max 1 g/dose), **THEN** repeat in 2 weeks

PEARLS
- May present with nocturnal perianal pruritus, abdominal pain, nausea, or vomiting
- Scotch tape applied to the perianal area can be examined microscopically for eggs
- Consider treatment of all household contacts
- Vacuum carpet, wash clothing, towels, and bedding in hot water
- Pyrantel pamoate is the recommended treatment in pregnant patients and is available as an over-the-counter preparation for ages ≥ 2 and older in U.S.

SCABIES/MITES

- Permethrin 5% cream: apply to entire body, wash off after 8–14 hrs, **THEN** repeat in 1 week (> 2 months old) if infestation persists
- Ivermectin 200 mcg/kg PO once, **THEN** repeat in 2 weeks (caution in pregnant/breastfeeding women and in children < 15 kg)
- Crotamiton 10% lotion: apply daily for 2 days (apply after bathing; not recommended for pediatric patients)

PEARLS
- Wash clothing and bedding in hot water, dry-clean, or place in airtight bag for 72 hrs
- Treat all close contacts
- Use oral and topical agents simultaneously for crusted scabies
- Ivermectin PO treatment should be first-line therapy for outbreaks in nursing homes and cohabitation facilities
- Consider antihistamines for pruritis

SEPSIS

Sepsis

- ▪ Life-threatening organ dysfunction caused by a dysregulated host response to infection
- ▪ Organ dysfunction should be identified by history, physical exam, laboratory findings, and clinical judgement
- ▪ Standardized early screening tools such as the Sequential [Sepsis-related] Organ Failure Assessment (SOFA) and qSOFA may improve sepsis recognition but are not sensitive enough to be used as the sole strategy for sepsis screening

Septic Shock

- ▪ A subset of sepsis in which particularly profound circulatory, cellular, and metabolic abnormalities are associated with a greater risk of mortality than with sepsis alone
- ▪ Defined as sepsis with cardiovascular dysfunction (spectrum that ranges from hypotension alone to refractory shock)

Initial Management

- ▪ Resuscitate patients with sepsis-induced hypoperfusion or septic shock
  - – Fluid resuscitation should be guided by dynamic measures (passive leg raise or a fluid bolus, using stroke volume (SV), stroke volume variation (SVV), pulse pressure variation (PPV), or echocardiography) over physical examination or static parameters alone
  - – Patients may benefit from 30 mL/kg of crystalloid within the first 3 hrs, but there is no prespecified volume that should be given
  - – Consider early peripheral vasopressor support coupled with volume expansion. There is no specific minimum fluid amount required before starting vasopressor support
  - – Continued IV fluid resuscitation (after initial resuscitation) should be guided by frequent assessments of hemodynamic status and patient response
  - – In patients with elevated lactate levels, resuscitation should be guided to decrease serum lactate

- Administer broad-spectrum antibiotics (shorter time frame is preferred but optimal timing remains to be determined)
  – Empiric broad-spectrum therapy against gram-positive and gram-negative bacteria according to local susceptibility should be administered in patients without a confirmed source
  – Targeted therapy according to source-specific guidelines should be started for patients with identified sources of infection
  – Specific treatment with anti-viral and anti-fungal therapy should be initiated in the ED for patients who may require additional coverage
- Blood cultures should be obtained prior to starting antimicrobial therapy but should not result in substantial delay in administering therapy
- When applicable, source control intervention should be implemented as soon as medically and logistically practical

Management of MAP < 65 mmHg despite initial fluid resuscitation

- Vasoactive medications
  – Norepinephrine = First line
  – **ADD** either epinephrine or vasopressin to norepinephrine if needed to reach target MAP
  – Consider adding vasopressin to decrease norepinephrine dosage
  – Consider dobutamine for persistent hypoperfusion despite adequate fluid loading and use of vasopressor agents
- Continued IV fluid resuscitation (after initial resuscitation) should be guided by frequent assessments of hemodynamic status
- Consider IV hydrocortisone (200 mg/day) if hemodynamic instability persists despite adequate fluid resuscitation and vasopressor therapy

Note: These recommendations do not fully encompass or strictly adhere to the CMS sepsis mandates

SEPSIS

BABESIOSIS

Common organism: *Babesia microti* (tick vector: *Ixodes scapularis*)

Mild (Parasitemia < 4%)
(Treatment duration: 7–10 days)
- Azithromycin 500 mg (Ⓟ 10 mg/kg) PO once, **THEN** 250 mg (Ⓟ 5 mg/kg) PO once daily **AND** atovaquone 750 mg (Ⓟ 20 mg/kg) PO two times daily

Severe (Parasitemia ≥ 4%)
(Treatment duration: 7–10 days)
- Azithromycin 500 mg (Ⓟ 10 mg/kg/day) IV **AND** atovaquone 750 mg (Ⓟ 20 mg/kg) PO two times daily
- Clindamycin 600 mg (Ⓟ 10 mg/kg) PO three times daily **AND** quinine 650 mg (Ⓟ 10 mg/kg) PO three times daily

PEARLS
- Consider Lyme disease, Rocky Mountain spotted fever, and ehrlichiosis/anaplasmosis in endemic areas
- Recommend consultation with ID
- Diagnosis preferred by Giemsa or Wright-stained thin blood smears. Acute babesiosis cannot be diagnosed by presence of babesia antibody because it can persist in blood for a year or longer
- Immunocompromised patients with severe disease require at least 6 weeks of therapy (2 weeks with negative blood smear)
- Indications for exchange transfusion: ≥ 10% parasitemia, hemoglobin < 10 g/dL, pulmonary, or hepatorenal impairment
- Common laboratory findings include anemia, thrombocytopenia, elevated lactate dehydrogenase, hyperbilirubinemia, and/or elevated transaminases
- 95% of cases: CT, MA, MN, NJ, NY, RI, WI

EHRLICHIOSIS/ANAPLASMOSIS

Organisms: *Ehrlichia chaffeensis, E. ewingii,* or *E. muris,* human monocytic ehrlichiosis (HME), *Anaplasma phagocytophilum,* human granulocytic anaplasmosis (HGA)
- Doxycycline 100 mg (Ⓟ 2.2 mg/kg) PO/IV two times daily for 3–5 days after fever resolves
- Pregnant: rifampin 300 mg PO two times daily for 3–5 days after fever resolves

PEARLS

- Treatment should be extended to 10 days for possible coinfection of Lyme disease
- Doxycycline is the recommended therapy for all ages and should not be delayed for laboratory testing in patients with suspected disease
- Common lab findings: leukopenia, thrombocytopenia, mildly elevated transaminases
- Most sensitive diagnostic testing is IFA (indirect fluorescent antibody assay)
- Recommend consultation with ID
- Treatment should be continued for 3–5 days after the fever resolves
- Consider Lyme disease, Rocky Mountain spotted fever, and babesiosis in endemic areas
- In 2021, Canada was forced to activate its crisis strategy for combatting an emergency shortage of maple syrup

LYME DISEASE

Common organism: *B. burgdorferi* (tick vector: *Ixodes ricinus* complex, animal reservoir: white footed mouse, white tailed deer)

Prophylaxis (ALL IDSA inclusion criteria should be met)
1) correct tick: identified as Ixodes, 2) correct time: > 36 hrs attached and/or engorged tick and < 72 hrs since removal, 3) correct location: endemic area = Northeast U.S., mid-Atlantic, some of the Midwest)

- Doxycycline 200 mg (ⓟ 4.4 mg/kg) PO once
- < 8 years old or pregnant, consider withholding prophylaxis and follow clinically for signs of infection

Erythema migrans or mild cardiac sequelae
(1st degree AV block < 300 msec)

- Doxycycline 100 mg (ⓟ 2.2 mg/kg) PO two times daily for 10–21 days
- Amoxicillin 500 mg (ⓟ 15 mg/kg) PO three times daily for 14–21 days
- Cefuroxime 500 mg (ⓟ 15 mg/kg) PO two times daily for 14–21 days
- Second-line for EM only: azithromycin 500 mg (ⓟ 10 mg/kg) PO once daily for 7 days

Serious cardiac disease
(1st degree AV block > 300 msec, 2nd or 3rd degree AV block, other dysrhythmias)
(Treatment duration: 14–21 days)

- Ceftriaxone 2 g (ⓟ 50–75 mg/kg) IV once daily
- Penicillin G 4M units (ⓟ 50,000 units/kg) IV six times daily
- Cefotaxime 2 g (ⓟ 50 mg/kg) IV three times daily

Neurologic disease

(Meningitis, radiculopathy, CN palsies, cognitive deficits)
(Treatment duration: 14–21 days)

- Ceftriaxone 2 g (P 50–75 mg/kg) IV once daily
- Penicillin G 4M units (P 50,000 units/kg) IV six times daily

Arthritis without neurologic sequelae

(Treatment duration: 28 days)

- Doxycycline 100 mg (P 2 mg/kg) PO two times daily
- Amoxicillin 500 mg (P 15 mg/kg) PO three times daily
- Cefuroxime 500 mg (P 15 mg/kg) PO two times daily

PEARLS

- Consider concomitant tick-borne diseases: babesiosis and anaplasmosis/ehrlichiosis
- The majority of patients with erythema migrans do not recall a tick bite and time to presentation of rash varies between 3–30 days
- Treatment not indicated for asymptomatic seropositive patients
- If necessary, consider penicillin desensitization for serious cardiac or neurologic disease
- Pregnant or breastfeeding: avoid doxycycline, use alternatives as above

MALARIA

CDC Malaria Hotline Main: 770-488-7788. After hours, weekends, and holidays call 770-488-7100 and page the CDC Malaria Branch Clinician

Common organisms: *P. falciparum, P. vivax, P. ovale, P. malariae, P. knowlesi*

Clinical presentation of uncomplicated malaria

- Symptoms are non-specific and commonly consist of fever, malaise, weakness, headache, myalgia, GI complaints, and chills
- Can be confused with a viral syndrome
- If a patient develops malaria while on chemoprophylaxis, that particular medication should not be used as part of the treatment regimen, and an alternative option should be selected

P. falciparum or species not identified, chloroquine-resistant or unknown resistance (all malarious regions, except those identified as chloroquine-sensitive, see PEARLS)

Adult—Any *ONE* of the following regimens

- Atovaquone/proguanil adult tab = 250 mg atovaquone/100 mg proguanil
  - 4 adult tabs PO once daily for 3 days

- Artemether/lumefantrine 1 tablet = 20 mg artemether/120 mg lumefantrine (standard adult dose is 4 tablets)
  - A 3-day treatment schedule with a total of 6 oral doses is recommended based on weight. The patient should receive the initial dose, followed by the second dose 8 hrs later, **THEN** 1 dose PO two times daily for the following 2 days
- Quinine sulfate 542 mg base (650 mg salt) PO three times daily for 3 or 7 days (*see PEARLS*) **PLUS:**
  - Doxycycline 100 mg PO two times daily for 7 days **OR**
  - Tetracycline 250 mg PO four times daily for 7 days **OR**
  - Clindamycin 7 mg base/kg/day PO three times daily for 7 days
- Mefloquine 684 mg base (750 mg salt) PO as initial dose, **THEN** 456 mg base (500 mg salt) PO 6–12 hrs after initial dose. Total dose = 1250 mg salt

Pediatric—Any *ONE* of the following regimens

- Atovaquone/proguanil adult tablet = 250 mg atovaquone/100 mg proguanil pediatric tablet = 62.5 mg atovaquone/25 mg proguanil
  - **5–8 kg:** 2 pediatric tablets PO once daily for 3 days
  - **9–10 kg:** 3 pediatric tablets PO once daily for 3 days
  - **11–20 kg:** 1 adult tablet PO once daily for 3 days
  - **21–30 kg:** 2 adult tablets PO once daily for 3 days
  - **31–40 kg:** 3 adult tablets PO once daily for 3 days
  - **> 40 kg:** 4 adult tablets PO once daily for 3 days
- Artemether/lumefantrine 1 tablet = 20 mg artemether/120 mg lumefantrine
  - A 3-day treatment schedule with a total of 6 oral doses is recommended for both adult and pediatric patients based on weight. The patient should receive the initial dose, followed by the second dose 8 hrs later, **THEN** 1 dose PO two times daily for the following 2 days
    - **5–14 kg:** 1 tablet per dose
    - **15–24 kg:** 2 tablets per dose
    - **25–35 kg:** 3 tablets per dose
    - **> 35 kg:** 4 tablets per dose
- Quinine sulfate: 8.3 mg base/kg (10 mg salt/kg) PO 3 times daily for 3 or 7 days (*see PEARLS*) **PLUS:**
  - Doxycycline 2.2 mg/kg PO two times daily for 7 days (not for < 8 y/o) **OR**
  - Tetracycline 6 mg/kg PO four times daily for 7 days (not for < 8 y/o) **OR**
  - Clindamycin 7 mg/kg PO three times daily for 7 days (for all ages)
- Mefloquine 13.7 mg base/kg (15 mg salt/kg) PO as initial dose, **THEN** 9.1 mg base/kg (10 mg salt/kg) PO 6–12 hrs after initial dose. Total dose = 25 mg salt/kg

ARTHROPOD-BORNE DISEASES AND PARASITIC INFECTIONS

P. malariae, P. knowlesi and *P. falciparum* or species not identified, chloroquine-sensitive

Adult

- Chloroquine phosphate 600 mg base (1 g salt) PO immediately, **THEN** 300 mg base (500 mg salt) PO at 6, 24, and 48 hours for a total dose of 1500 mg (2500 mg salt)
- Hydroxychloroquine 620 mg base (800 mg salt) PO immediately, **THEN** 310 mg base (400 mg salt) PO at 6, 24, and 48 hours for a total dose of 1,550 mg base (2000 mg salt)

Pediatric

- Chloroquine phosphate 10 mg base/kg PO immediately, **THEN** 5 mg base/kg PO at 6, 24, and 48 hours (total dose 25 mg base/kg)
- Hydroxychloroquine 10 mg base/kg immediately, **THEN** 5 mg/base/kg PO at 6, 24, and 48 hours (total dose of 25 mg base/kg)

P. vivax and *P. ovale*, Chloroquine-sensitive

(except *P. vivax* in Papua New Guinea and Indonesia, see next section)

Adult

- Chloroquine phosphate 600 mg base (1 g salt) PO immediately, **THEN** 300 mg base (500 mg salt) PO at 6, 24 and 48 hours for a total dose 1500 mg (2500 mg salt) **AND** primaquine phosphate 30 mg base PO once daily for 14 days
- Hydroxychloroquine 620 mg base (800 mg salt) PO immediately, **THEN** 310 mg base (400 mg salt) PO at 6, 24, and 48 hours for a total dose of 1550 mg base (2000 mg salt) **AND** primaquine phosphate 30 mg base PO once daily for 14 days

Pediatric

- Chloroquine phosphate 10 mg base/kg PO immediately, **THEN** 5 mg base/kg PO at 6, 24, and 48 hours (total dose 25 mg base/kg) **AND** primaquine phosphate 0.5 mg base/kg PO once daily for 14 days
- Hydroxychloroquine 10 mg base/kg immediately, **THEN** 5 mg/base/kg PO at 6, 24, and 48 hours (total dose of 25 mg base/kg) **AND** primaquine phosphate 0.5 mg base/kg PO once daily for 14 days

ARTHROPOD-BORNE DISEASES AND PARASITIC INFECTIONS

P. vivax, Chloroquine-resistant
(Papua New Guinea and Indonesia)

Adult
Any *ONE* of the following regimens
- Quinine sulfate 542 mg base (650 mg salt) PO three times daily for 3 or 7 days (see *PEARLS*) **AND** primaquine phosphate 30 mg base PO once daily for 14 days **PLUS:**
  - Doxycycline 100 mg PO two times daily for 7 days **OR**
  - Tetracycline 250 mg PO four times daily for 7 days
- Atovaquone/proguanil 4 adult tabs PO once daily for 3 days **AND** primaquine phosphate 30 mg base PO once daily for 14 days
- Mefloquine 684 mg base (750 mg salt) PO as initial dose, **THEN** 456 mg base (500 mg salt) PO 6–12 hrs after initial dose. Total dose = 1250 mg salt **AND** primaquine phosphate 30 mg base PO once daily for 14 days

Pediatric
Any *ONE* of the 3 following regimens
- Mefloquine 13.7 mg base/kg (15 mg salt/kg) PO as initial dose, **THEN** 9.1 mg base/kg (10 mg salt/kg) PO 6–12 hrs after initial dose. Total dose = 25 mg salt/kg **AND** primaquine phosphate 0.5 mg base/kg PO once daily for 14 days
- Quinine sulfate 8.3 mg base/kg (10 mg salt/kg) PO 3 times daily for 3 or 7 days (see *PEARLS*) **AND** primaquine phosphate 0.5 mg base/kg PO once daily for 14 days **AND** doxycycline 2.2 mg/kg PO two times daily for 7 days (Ⓟ not for < 8 years old)
- Atovaquone/proguanil adult tablet = 250 mg atovaquone/100 mg proguanil pediatric tablet = 62.5 mg atovaquone/25 mg proguanil
  - **5–8 kg:** 2 pediatric tablets PO once daily for 3 days
  - **9–10 kg:** 3 pediatric tablets PO once daily for 3 days
  - **11–20 kg:** 1 adult tablet PO once daily for 3 days
  - **21–30 kg:** 2 adult tablets PO once daily for 3 days
  - **31–40 kg:** 3 adult tablets PO once daily for 3 days
  - **> 40 kg:** 4 adult tablets PO once daily for 3 days

Pregnant
Chloroquine-sensitive
- Chloroquine phosphate 600 mg base (1 g salt) PO **THEN** 300 mg base (500 mg salt) PO at 6, 24, and 48 hours. Total dose 1500 mg (2500 mg salt)
- Hydroxychloroquine 620 mg base (800 mg salt) PO immediately, **THEN** 310 mg base (400 mg salt) PO at 6, 24, and 48 hours after the initial dose. Total dose = 1550 mg base (2000 mg salt)

Chloroquine-resistant *P. falciparum* and *P. vivax*

- ◼ Quinine sulfate 542 mg base (650 mg salt) PO three times daily for 3 or 7 days (see *PEARLS*) **AND** clindamycin 600 mg PO three times daily for 7 days
- ◼ Mefloquine 684 mg base (750 mg salt) PO as initial dose, **THEN** 456 mg base (500 mg salt) PO 6–12 hrs after initial dose. Total dose = 1250 mg salt
- ◼ **For chloroquine-resistant *P. falciparum* ONLY, consider:**
  - — Artemether/lumefantrine 1 tablet = 20 mg artemether/120 mg lumefantrine. A 3-day treatment schedule with a total of 6 oral doses (24 tabs). The patient should receive initial dose (4 tabs) , followed by second dose (4 tabs) 8 hrs later, **THEN** 1 dose (4 tabs) PO two times daily for the following two days. Can be used during the 2nd and 3rd trimester (limited data in 1st trimester)

Clinical Presentation of Complicated (Severe) Malaria (usually because of *P. falciparum*)

Defined by one or more of the following: impaired consciousness/coma, renal failure, pulmonary edema, shock, jaundice, disseminated intravascular coagulation, parasitemia of > 5%, severe normocytic anemia (Hgb < 7), ARDS, hemoglobinuria, and/or convulsions

- ◼ IV artesunate recommended for use in infants, children, and pregnant women
- ◼ **Clindamycin and doxycycline not recommended as slow-acting and not recommended as monotherapy**

Artesunate

- ◼ **Adults and children ≥ 20 kg**: 2.4 mg/kg IV at 0 hour, 12 hrs, 24 hrs, and 48 hrs
- ◼ **Children < 20 kg**: 3.0 mg/kg IV at 0 hour, 12 hrs, 24 hrs, and 48 hrs
- ◼ While waiting for IV artesunate, choose **ONE** of the following choices:
  - — **Artemether/lumefantrine**: 1 tablet = 20 mg artemether/120 mg lumefantrine. The patient should receive the initial dose (4 tabs), followed by the second dose (4 tabs) 8 hrs later if still needed. Consider via nasogastric tube if not able to take oral medications
  - — **Atovaquone/proguanil**: Adult (250 mg atovaquone/100 mg proguanil) and pediatric (62.5 mg atovaquone/25 mg proguanil) formulations are available. **Adults:** 4 adult tablets as 1 dose. Consider via nasogastric tube if not able to take oral medications
  - — **Quinine sulfate: Adults:** 650 mg (salt) PO three times daily. **Children:** 10 mg (salt)/kg PO three times daily. Consider via nasogastric tube if not able to take oral medications
- ◼ After the course of IV artesunate is completed, choose **ONE** of the following:

- **Artemether/lumefantrine:** 1 tablet = 20 mg artemether and 120 mg lumefantrine. A 3-day treatment schedule with a total of 6 oral doses as follows: initial dose, second dose 8 hrs later, then 1 dose twice daily for the following 2 days (Dosing as recommended by CDC)
- **Atovaquone/proguanil:** One dose daily for 3 days (Dosing as recommended by CDC)
- **Doxycycline: Adults:** 100 mg PO two times per day for 7 days. **Children** (≥ 8 years): 2 mg/kg PO two times per day for 7 days
  - Children < 8 years old or pregnant women should instead receive clindamycin 10 mg/kg PO three times daily for 7 days
  - Access CDC for pediatric dosing recommendations

PEARLS

- Suspect in any febrile patient returning from the tropics
- CDC encourages reporting all cases using Malaria Case Report Form: www.cdc.gov/malaria/report.html
- In non-endemic areas, treatment for malaria should not be initiated until diagnosis is confirmed. "Presumptive" treatment should only be used for extreme circumstances
- For country-specific resistance patterns and country-specific species check CDC website at www.cdc.gov/malaria/travelers/country_table
- Call CDC with any failure of treatment
- Thick and thin blood smears every 12–24 hrs for a total of 3 sets to make diagnosis; one negative smear is not enough to rule out suspected malaria
- Primaquine can cause hemolytic anemia in persons with G6PD deficiency
- Mefloquine noted to cause neuropsychiatric reactions in some patients
- RBC exchange transfusion should be considered for the most severe cases such as parasite density > 10%, ARDS, renal complications, or cerebral malaria
- Pregnant women diagnosed with severe malaria should be aggressively treated with parenteral therapy; tetracycline, doxycycline, and primaquine are contraindicated
- In 2018, the FDA approved tafenoquine to prevent *P. vivax* malaria relapse as single-dose therapy

NEUROCYSTICERCOSIS

Common organism: *Taenia solium* (pork tapeworm)
- 1-2 viable cysts: albendazole 7.5 mg/kg PO two times daily (max 1200 mg/day) with food for 10 days in consultation with ID
- > 2 viable cysts: albendazole 7.5 mg/kg PO two times daily (max 1200 mg/day) **PLUS** praziquantel 5 mg/kg PO three times daily for 10 days in consultation with ID

PEARLS
- Initiation of anti-parasitic therapy is rarely a medical emergency
- Calcified cysts do not require antihelminthic therapy
- Adjuvant therapies include corticosteroids and anti-convulsants; hydrocephalus may require surgical consultation
- Antiparasitic therapy initiation may acutely worsen neurological symptoms and is not recommended for patients with cerebral edema or elevated ICP

ROCKY MOUNTAIN SPOTTED FEVER

Common organism: *Rickettsia rickettsii*

(Treatment duration: for at least 3 days after the fever subsides and until evidence of clinical improvement is noted, typically for a minimum of 5–7 days)

- Doxycycline 100 mg (Ⓟ 2.2 mg/kg) PO/IV two times daily

PEARLS
- Treatment is based on clinical suspicion and should begin before laboratory confirmation
- For critically ill patients, consider a loading dose of doxycycline 200 mg IV two times daily for 3 days
- Doxycycline is the drug of choice for children; risk of dental staining is minimal with one course of doxycycline
- Pregnant: Current evidence suggests short-term doxycycline therapy is unlikely to pose teratogenic effects and is the drug of choice after a discussion of risks and benefits
- Prophylaxis following tick bite to prevent infection is not recommended

ARTHROPOD-BORNEDISEASES AND PARASITIC INFECTIONS

CEPHALOSPORINS
- Ceftriaxone should not be administered to any patient < 28 days old because it has been shown to cause increased hyperbilirubinemia and precipitation of calcium into lungs and kidneys of neonates
- Use has been shown to be associated with angioedema, thrombocytopenia, nonconvulsive status epilepticus, hemolytic anemia, eosinophilia, hepatitis, and increased risk for superinfections
- Increases risk of thrush, yeast infections, and other fungal infections

LINEZOLID
- Common reactions
  - Lactic acidosis
  - Altered taste perception
- Use with caution with SSRIs because of increased risk of serotonin syndrome; contraindicated with use of MAOIs and meperidine
- Caution with tyramine-containing foods (aged cheese, beer, wine, smoked meats) because of risk of precipitating hypertensive crisis
- Prolonged use associated with thrombocytopenia, myelosuppression, peripheral and optic neuropathy

METRONIDAZOLE
- Common reactions
  - GI upset
  - Confusion
  - Ataxia
  - Metallic taste
- Traditionally warn patients of potential alcohol interaction within 72 hrs of administration to avoid disulfiram-like reaction; however, there is no evidence to support this
- Prolonged use associated with aseptic meningitis, seizures, neuropathies

NITROFURANTOIN
- Efficacy limited if CrCl < 30 mL/min
- May cause hemolytic anemia; do not use in patients with G6PD deficiency, infants < 1 month old, or pregnant patients near term
- **AVOID** during first trimester unless there is no therapeutic alternative
- **AVOID** in patients > 36 weeks gestation because of increased risk of neonatal hemolytic anemia
- Warn patients that their urine may turn brown

PENICILLINS

- Use is associated with thrombocytopenia, hemolytic anemia, and seizures, especially at high doses in patients with renal failure

QUINOLONES

- U.S. boxed warnings
  - Myasthenia gravis exacerbation
  - Peripheral neuropathy
  - CNS effects)
  - Tendonitis/tendon rupture
- Give at least 1 hour before or 2 hours after antacids or other drug products containing calcium, iron, or zinc
- May decrease elimination of methylxanthines (eg, theophylline and caffeine)
- May cause a lower seizure threshold (especially if given with NSAIDs)
- May cause QT prolongation
- Associated with hypo/hyperglycemia
- Data suggest an increased risk of aortic dissection/aneurysm and should be used cautiously in those at already increased risk

TRIMETHOPRIM/SULFAMETHOXAZOLE (TMP/SMX)

- Common reactions
  - Rash
  - Photosensitivity
- Sulfonamides have a high incidence of hypersensitivity reactions
- Patients should be advised to maintain adequate hydration due to potential transient elevation of creatinine and potassium
- TMP/SMX is contraindicated in pregnancy due to its interference with folic acid metabolism and is excreted in breast milk so is generally advisable not to use if breastfeeding.
- **AVOID during first trimester** unless there is no therapeutic alternative
- **AVOID** in patients > 36 weeks gestation due to increased risk of neonatal hemolytic anemia (nitrofurantoin) or kernicterus (sulfonamides)
- **AVOID** in patients > age 65 years who are also on an ACE inhibitor or ARB
- Do not give to patients with G6PD deficiency, anemia due to folate deficiency, history of drug induced ITP, or infants < 4 weeks
- Use has been shown to cause dose-dependent blood dyscrasias including thrombocytopenia, megaloblastic anemia, and neutropenia

TETRACYCLINES
- Common reactions
  - Pill esophagitis
  - GI upset
  - Photosensitivity
- May cause tooth enamel hypoplasia and tissue hyperpigmentation in children < 8 years old
  - More common with long-term use
  - Observed with repeated short courses
  - Use in children when benefits outweigh risk
- Relatively contraindicated in pregnancy and breastfeeding: pregnancy class D
- Potentiates digoxin levels
- Avoid antacids, dairy products, and iron within 2 hrs of ingestion
- To reduce the risk of esophageal injury, take on an empty stomach with a full glass of water and do not lay flat for 30 min
- Can cause skin photosensitivity; intense sunlight exposure should be avoided
- Ingesting expired tetracyclines can cause Fanconi syndrome

VANCOMYCIN
- May cause infusion-related reactions — flushing, erythema, and pruritus, usually affecting the upper body, neck, and face. This is an infusion rate-related side effect and not a true allergy
- Can be nephrotoxic and requires renal dosing
- Prolonged use is associated with neutropenia and increased risk for superinfections

WARFARIN AND ANTIBIOTICS
- Many antibiotics can affect INR and warrant more frequent measurement
- Common medications that
  - Decrease INR: dicloxacillin, griseofulvin, nafcillin, and rifampin
  - Increase INR: azole antifungals, cephalosporins, chloramphenicol, isoniazid, macrolides, metronidazole, quinolones, sulfonamides

PROLONGED QT AND ANTIBIOTICS
- Common antimicrobials that prolong the QT interval: azole antifungals, macrolides, pentamidine, fluoroquinolones, TMP/SMX, and antimalarials

ANTICONVULSANTS AND ANTIBIOTICS
- Multiple antibiotics interfere with the metabolism of anticonvulsants, especially phenytoin. Review potential drug interactions before prescribing new antibiotics to patients taking anticonvulsants

IDEAL BODY WEIGHT CHART

Height (in)	Height (cm)	Male Ideal body weight (kg)	Female Ideal body weight (kg)
60	152.4	50	46
61	154.94	52	48
62	157.48	55	50
63	160.02	57	52
64	162.56	59	55
65	165.1	62	57
66	167.64	64	59
67	170.18	66	62
68	172.72	68	64
69	175.26	71	66
70	177.8	73	69
71	180.34	75	71
72	182.88	78	73
73	185.42	80	75
74	187.96	82	78
75	190.5	85	80
76	193.04	87	82
77	195.58	89	85
78	198.12	91	87
79	200.66	94	89
80	203.2	96	92

Drugs to consider using IBW:

- Acyclovir (for severe infections such as HSV encephalitis, consider using adjusted body weight)
- Colistin
- Ethambutol
- Pyrazinamide
- Aminoglycosides
  - Aminoglycoside dosing weight = ideal body weight (IBW)
  - Use actual body weight (ABW) if it is less than IBW
  - If morbidly obese (> 20% over ideal body weight), use adjusted body weight (AdjBW)
    - AdjBW = 0.4 (ABW-IBW) + IBW

PENICILLIN/CEPHALOSPORIN ALLERGY ALGORITHM

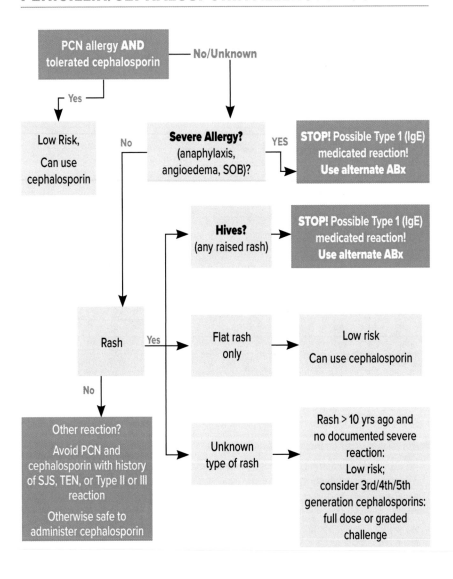

Cephalosporins are the preferred empiric antibiotic choice for many infectious diseases. Patients with a labeled penicillin allergy are 3 times more likely to have an adverse outcome related to antibiotic therapy. Time spent to do a thorough allergy history can go a long way. **Although 10% of the population reports a PCN allergy, 90% of patients can tolerate. The true risk of anaphylaxis to penicillin is 0.01%—and 80% of patients will lose their Type (igE) medicated reaction (eg, hives, anaphylaxis, SOB) after 10 years.**

CEPHALOSPORIN REFERENCE

1st Generation Cephalosporins		
Generic	**Trade**	**Route**
Cefadroxil	Duricef®	PO
Cephalexin	Bio-Cef®, Keflex®, Keftab®	PO
Cefazolin	Ancef®	IM/IV
2nd Generation Cephalosporins		
Generic	**Trade**	**Route**
Cefaclor	Ceclor®, Raniclor®	PO
Cefprozil	Cefzil®	PO
Cefuroxime axetil	(generic)	PO
Cefuroxime sodium	Zinacef®	IM/IV
Cefoxitin	Mefoxin®	IM/IV
Cefotetan	Cefotan®	IM/IV
3rd Generation Cephalosporins		
Generic	**Trade**	**Route**
Cefdinir	Omnicef®	PO
Cefditoren	Spectracef®	PO
Ceftibuten	Cedax®	PO
Cefixime	Suprax®	PO
Cefpodoxime proxetil	Vantin®	PO
Ceftazidime	Tazicef®, Fortaz®	IV
Ceftazidime/avibactam	Avycaz® Zavicefta®	IV
Ceftriaxone	Rocephin®	IM/IV
4th Generation Cephalosporins		
Generic	**Trade**	**Route**
Cefepime	Maxipime®	IV
5th Generation Cephalosporins		
Generic	**Trade**	**Route**
Ceftaroline	Teflaro®	IV
Extended Spectrum Cephalosporins		
Generic	**Trade**	**Route**
Cefiderocol	Fetroja®	IV
Ceftolozane/tazobactam	Zerbaxa®	IV
Cefoperazone/sulbactam	Cefobid®	IM/IV

PREGNANCY/LACTATION SAFETY TABLE

Antibiotic	Pregnancy Class	Lactation Safety
NOTE: Assigning classes based on safety is complex and currently being re-evaluated by the FDA. Guidance will be updated in the EMRA Antibiotic Guide app as it becomes available.		
Acyclovir	B	S
Ampicillin	B	PS
Ampicillin/Sulbactam	B	PS
Amoxicillin	B	S
Amoxicillin/Clavulanate	B	PS
Amphotericin B	B	U
Azithromycin	B	PN
Aztreonam	B	PS
Cefadroxil	B	PS
Cefazolin	B	S
Cefepime	B	PS
Cefotetan	B	U
Cefpodoxime/Cefdinir	B	PS
Ceftazidime/Avibactam	B	U
Ceftolozane/Tazobactam	B	U
Cefuroxime/Ceftriaxone	B	PS
Cephalexin	B	S
Chloramphenicol	C	PN
Chloroquine phosphate	C	PS
Ciprofloxacin	C	U
Clarithromycin	C	PN
Clindamycin	B	PN
Clotrimazole	C	PN
Dalbavancin	C	U
Dapsone	C	PN
Daptomycin	B	U
Dicloxacillin	B	U
Doxycycline	D	PN
Ertapenem	B	U
Famciclovir	B	U
Fidaxomicin	B	U
Fluconazole	C (single dose), D	U
Fosfomycin	B	U
Ganciclovir	C	N

Antibiotic	Pregnancy Class	Lactation Safety
Gentamicin	D	PS
Griseofulvin	X	U
Hydroxychloroquine	C	PS
Imipenem/Cilastatin	C	PS
Ivermectin	C	U
Ketoconazole	C	U
Levofloxacin	C	PN
Linezolid	C	U
Meropenem	B	U
Metronidazole	B	U
Miconazole	C	PN
Minocycline	D	PN
Moxifloxacin	C	U
Nafcillin	B	PS
Nitrofurantoin	B, D (3rd trimester)	PS
Nystatin	C	S
Oxacillin	B	U
Penicillin	B	S
Piperacillin/Tazobactam	B	PS
Praziquantel	B	PS
Terbinafine	B	U
Tetracycline	D	U
TMP/SMX	D	PN
Tobramycin	D	U
Valacyclovir	B	PS
Valganciclovir	C	PN
Vancomycin	B	PN
Voriconazole	D	U

Lactation Safety	
S	safe
N	not safe
PS	prob safe
PN	prob not safe
U	uncertain

Pregnancy Class	
A	Controlled human studies show no risk
B	Animal studies show no risk of adverse fetal effects, but human studies unavailable
C	Animal studies show adverse fetal effects, but no controlled human studies
D	Positive evidence of human fetal risk; maternal benefit may outweigh fetal risk
X	Contraindicated: Postive evidence of serious fetal abnormalities in humans

ANTIBIOTIC COVERAGE TABLE

Name	Gram Positive	Gram Negative	Anaerobe	*Pseudomonas*	MRSA	Atypical bacteria
Amoxicillin/ Clavulanate, Ampicillin/ Sulbactam	+	+	+			
Ampicillin, Amoxicillin	+					
Azithromycin	+/-					+
Aztreonam		+		+		
Cefazolin, Cephalexin	+	+				
Cefepime	+	+		+		
Cefoxitin, Cefotetan	+	+	+/-			
Ceftriaxone	+	+				
Ciprofloxacin		+		+		+
Clindamycin	+		+		+/-	
Ertapenem	+	+	+			
Gentamicin	synergy	+		+		
Imipenem/ cilastatin, meropenem	+	+	+	+		
Levofloxacin	+	+		+		+
Linezolid	+				+	
Metronidazole			+			
Moxifloxacin	+	+	+			+
Oxacillin	+					
Penicillin	+		+/-			
Piperacillin/ tazobactam	+	+	+	+		
Tetracyclines	+	+			+	+
TMP/SMX	+	+			+	
Vancomycin	+				+	

ANTIBIOTIC COST TABLE

Medication	Cost	Medication	Cost	Medication	Cost
Abacavir	$$$$$	Daptomycin	$$$$$	Moxifloxacin	$$$
Acyclovir	$	Dicloxacillin	$$	Nafcillin	$$
Albendazole	$$$$$	Doxycycline	$$	Nitrofurantoin	$$
Amikacin	$$$	Emtricitabine/Tenofovir	$$$$$	Nystatin	$
Ampicillin	$	Ertapenem	$$$$	Ofloxacin	$$
Ampicillin/Sulbactam	$$	Erythromycin	$$$$$	Oritavancin	$$$$$
Amoxicillin	$	Ethambutol	$$$	Oseltamivir	$$$
Amoxicillin/Clavulanate	$$$	Famciclovir	$$$	Oxacillin	$
Amphotericin B	$$$$	Fidaxomicin	$$$$$	Penicillin	$-$$$
Atovaquone	$$$$$	Fluconazole	$	Pentamidine	$$$$
Azithromycin	$	Flucytosine	$$$$$	Piperacillin/Tazobactam	$$
Aztreonam	$$$$	Fosfomycin	$$$	Praziquantel	$$$$$
Caspofungin	$$$$$	Ganciclovir	$$$$$	Primaquine	$$
Cefadroxil	$$$	Gemifloxacin	$$	Pyrantel	$
Cefazolin	$$	Gentamicin	$$	Pyrazinamide	$$$$
Cefepime	$$	Griseofulvin	$$$	Quinine	$$$$
Cefpodoxime, Cefdinir	$$$$	Hydroxychloroquine	$$	Ribavirin	$$$$$
Ceftaroline	$$$$$	Imipenem/Cilastatin	$$$	Rifabutin	$$$$$
Ceftazidime	$$	Isoniazid	$	Rifampin	$$$
Ceftazidime/Avibactam	$$$$$	Itraconazole	$$$$	Ritonavir	$$$$$
Ceftolozane/Tazobactam	$$$$	Ivermectin	$	Streptomycin	$$$$$
Ceftriaxone	$$	Ketoconazole	$$	Telavancin	$$$$$
Cefuroxime	$$$	Lamivudine/Zidovudine	$$$$	Terbinafine	$$
Cephalexin	$	Levofloxacin	$$	Tetracycline	$$$$$
Chloroquine phosphate	$$$$	Linezolid	$$$	Tigecycline	$$$$$
Ciprofloxacin	$$	Mefloquine	$$	Trimethoprim/Sulfamethoxazole	$
Clarithromycin	$$$$$	Meropenem	$$$$	Tobramycin	$
Clindamycin	$$	Metronidazole	$	Valacyclovir	$$
Dalbavancin	$$$$$	Miconazole	$	Valganciclovir	$$$$$
Dapsone	$$	Minocycline	$$$$	Vancomycin	$$$$

LEGEND

Cost

$ = < $25	$$$ = $50–$99	$$$$$ = >$200
$$ = $25–$49	$$$$ = $100–$199	

COMMON PEDIATRIC DOSING

Approximate Pediatric ABx Dosing Medication (per dose)	Strength mg/tsp	Freq	Weight in kgt								
			5	6.5	8	9	10	11	13	15	19
Amoxicillin (high dose): 40-45 mg/kg	200/tsp	2x/day	1	1.25	1.75	2	2	2.25	2.75	3	4
	250/tsp	2x/day	3/4	1.25	1.5	1.5	1.75	1.75	2.25	2.5	3.25
	400/tsp	2x/day	1/2	3/4	3/4	1	1	1.25	1.25	1.5	2
Amoxicillin/Clavulanate or Amoxicillin (25 mg/kg)	125/tsp	2x/day	1	1.25	1.5	1.75	1.75	2	2.25	2.75	3.5
	200/tsp	2x/day	1/2	3/4	1	1	1.25	1.25	1.5	1.75	2.25
	250/tsp	2x/day	1/2	1/2	3/4	3/4	1	1	1.25	1.25	1.75
	400/tsp	2x/day	1/4	1/2	1/2	1/2	3/4	3/4	3/4	1	1
Amox/Clav ES (45 mg/kg)	600/tsp	2x/day	3/8	1/2	1/2	3/4	3/4	3/4	1	1.25	1.5
Azithromycin (5 mg/kg) (5-day course; double dose on Day 1)	100/tsp	daily	—	—	1/2	1/2	1/2	1/2	3/4	3/4	1
	200/tsp	daily	—	—	1/4	1/4	1/4	1/4	1/3	1/2	1/2
Cefaclor (15-20 mg/kg)	125/tsp	2x/day	3/4	1	1.25	1.5	1.5	1.75	2	2.5	3
	250/tsp	2x/day	1/3	1/2	3/4	3/4	3/4	1	1	1.25	1.5
Cefdinir (15 mg/kg)	125/tsp	daily	—	—	1	1	1	1.25	1.5	1.75	2
Cefixime (8 mg/kg)	100/tsp	daily	1/2	1/2	3/4	3/4	3/4	1	1	1.25	1.5
Cefuroxime (10-15 mg/kg)	125/tsp	2x/day	—	3/4	3/4	1	1	1	1.5	1.75	2.25
Cephalexin (10-15 mg/kg)	125/tsp	4x/day	—	1/2	3/4	3/4	1	1	1.25	1.5	1.75
	250/tsp	4x/day	—	1/4	1/4	1/2	1/2	1/2	3/4	3/4	1
Nitrofurantoin (1-2 mg/kg)	25/tsp	4x/day	1/4	1/2	1/2	1/2	1/2	3/4	3/4	3/4	1
TMP/SMX (4 mg/kg)	40/200/tsp	2x/day	1/2	3/4	1	1	1	1.25	1.5	1.5	2

INDEX

2e7b09e8-77b2-4dd4-b2a9-6ba3ccde3b21R01